Tumors
of the
Serosal Membranes

Atlas
of
Tumor Pathology

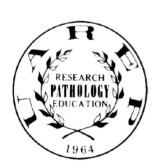

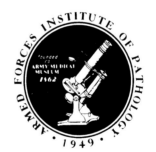

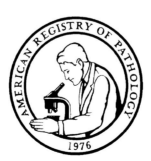

ATLAS OF TUMOR PATHOLOGY

Third Series
Fascicle 15

TUMORS OF THE SEROSAL MEMBRANES

by

HECTOR BATTIFORA, M.D.
Chairman, Division of Pathology
City of Hope National Medical Center
Duarte, California

W. T. ELLIOTT McCAUGHEY, M.D., F.R.C.P. (C)
Clinical Professor of Pathology
University of Ottawa
Ottawa, Canada

Published by the
ARMED FORCES INSTITUTE OF PATHOLOGY
Washington, D.C.

Under the Auspices of
UNIVERSITIES ASSOCIATED FOR RESEARCH AND EDUCATION IN PATHOLOGY, INC.
Bethesda, Maryland
1995

Accepted for Publication
1994

Available from the American Registry of Pathology
Armed Forces Institute of Pathology
Washington, D.C. 20306-6000
ISSN 0160-6344
ISBN 1-881041-19-0

ATLAS OF TUMOR PATHOLOGY

EDITOR
JUAN ROSAI, M.D.
Department of Pathology
Memorial Sloan-Kettering Cancer Center
New York, New York 10021-6007

ASSOCIATE EDITOR
LESLIE H. SOBIN, M.D.
Armed Forces Institute of Pathology
Washington, D.C. 20306-6000

EDITORS' NOTE

The Atlas of Tumor Pathology has a long and distinguished history. It was first conceived at a Cancer Research Meeting held in St. Louis in September 1947 as an attempt to standardize the nomenclature of neoplastic diseases. The first series was sponsored by the National Academy of Sciences-National Research Council. The organization of this Sisyphean effort was entrusted to the Subcommittee on Oncology of the Committee on Pathology, and Dr. Arthur Purdy Stout was the first editor-in-chief. Many of the illustrations were provided by the Medical Illustration Service of the Armed Forces Institute of Pathology, the type was set by the Government Printing Office, and the final printing was done at the Armed Forces Institute of Pathology (hence the colloquial appellation "AFIP Fascicles"). The American Registry of Pathology purchased the Fascicles from the Government Printing Office and sold them virtually at cost. Over a period of 20 years, approximately 15,000 copies each of nearly 40 Fascicles were produced. The worldwide impact that these publications have had over the years has largely surpassed the original goal. They quickly became among the most influential publications on tumor pathology ever written, primarily because of their overall high quality but also because their low cost made them easily accessible to pathologists and other students of oncology the world over.

Upon completion of the first series, the National Academy of Sciences-National Research Council handed further pursuit of the project over to the newly created Universities Associated for Research and Education in Pathology (UAREP). A second series was started, generously supported by grants from the AFIP, the National Cancer Institute, and the American Cancer Society. Dr. Harlan I. Firminger became the editor-in-chief and was succeeded by Dr. William H. Hartmann. The second series Fascicles were produced as bound volumes instead of loose leaflets. They featured a more comprehensive coverage of the subjects, to the extent that the Fascicles could no longer be regarded as "atlases" but rather as monographs describing and illustrating in detail the tumors and tumor-like conditions of the various organs and systems.

Once the second series was completed, with a success that matched that of the first, UAREP and AFIP decided to embark on a third series. A new editor-in-chief and an associate editor were selected, and a distinguished editorial board was appointed. The mandate for the third series remains the same as for the previous ones, i.e., to oversee the production of an eminently practical publication with surgical pathologists as its primary audience, but also aimed at other workers in oncology. The main purposes of this series are to promote a consistent, unified, and biologically sound nomenclature; to guide the surgical pathologist in the diagnosis of the various tumors and tumor-like lesions; and to provide relevant histogenetic, pathogenetic, and clinicopathologic information on these entities. Just as the second series included data obtained from ultrastructural (and, in the more recent Fascicles, immunohistochemical) examination, the third series will, in addition, incorporate pertinent information obtained with the newer molecular biology techniques. As in the past, a continuous attempt will be made to correlate, whenever possible, the nomenclature used in the Fascicles with that proposed by the World Health Organization's International Histological Classification of Tumors. The format of the third series has been changed in order to incorporate additional items and to ensure a consistency of style throughout. Close cooperation between the various authors and their respective liaisons from the editorial board will be emphasized to minimize unnecessary repetition and discrepancies in the text and illustrations.

To its everlasting credit, the participation and commitment of the AFIP to this venture is even more substantial and encompassing than in previous series. It now extends to virtually all scientific, technical, and financial aspects of the production.

The task confronting the organizations and individuals involved in the third series is even more daunting than in the preceding efforts because of the ever-increasing complexity of the matter at hand. It is hoped that this combined effort—of which, needless to say, that represented by the authors is first and foremost—will result in a series worthy of its two illustrious predecessors and will be a suitable introduction to the tumor pathology of the twenty-first century.

Juan Rosai, M.D.
Leslie H. Sobin, M.D.

PREFACE AND ACKNOWLEDGMENTS

Though physicians have detected fluid in the serous cavities and performed paracentesis since ancient times, involvement of the serous membranes by disease, distinct from processes primarily or predominantly affecting the parenchyma of underlying organs, was not clearly appreciated until the nineteenth century. Subsequent progress in clinical and laboratory medicine led to recognition that the tunica serosae may be involved by various types of inflammatory and reactive processes and tumors. Early on a controversy developed, which was protracted, concerning the status of malignant primary tumors, especially those thought to arise from the lining cells (mesothelium) of the serous membranes. Only within the past four or five decades has the existence of a malignant tumor of mesothelial cells (malignant mesothelioma) as an entity been generally accepted, and even today the varied histologic characteristics of malignant mesothelioma and its pathologic overlap with other neoplasms (sarcomas as well as adenocarcinomas) continue to complicate differentiation of this tumor from metastatic tumor.

Since 1960, interest in the accurate diagnosis and classification of serosal neoplasms has been stimulated greatly by evidence of an increased prevalence of diffuse malignant mesothelioma in persons exposed to asbestos. Most diffuse malignant mesotheliomas, in fact, appear to be caused by asbestos. This has given pathologic investigation and classification of primary malignant serosal neoplasms important epidemiologic and socioeconomic connotations, though, as yet, limited therapeutic significance. At the same time there has also been wider recognition of types of mesothelioma with unusual microscopic features or behavioral patterns and greater knowledge of the characteristics of localized fibrous tumors of sub-mesothelial origin. In addition, the remarkable range of metaplasias, pseudotumors, and low-grade tumors involving serous membrane, especially the peritoneum in females, has attracted increasing interest. Additionally, in recent years there has been a rapid growth in the application of immunohistochemistry to assist in the diagnosis of serosal neoplasms. These developments have led to rapid expansion of knowledge of serosal neoplasms and make it timely that the Second Series Fascicle of the Atlas of Tumor Pathology (Fascicle 20) entitled "Tumors and Pseudotumors of the Serous Membrane" be updated.

The authors are extremely grateful to the many pathologists in North America and abroad who over the years have referred interesting or otherwise problematic material to the institutions and panels with which they have been associated, who have permitted us to use their material for illustrative purposes, and who have provided follow-up information. We would also like to thank the following laboratory staff: Parula Mehta and Rosalba Tamayo in Duarte and Constance Clark in Ottawa.

We would also like to acknowledge the contribution of Dr. Jacob Churg and the late Dr. Milton Kannerstein both of whom played a major role in initiating and developing the Second Series Fascicle.

Hector Battifora, M.D.
W.T. Elliott McCaughey, M.D., F.R.C.P. (C)

TUMORS OF THE SEROSAL MEMBRANES

Contents

TUMORS OF THE SEROSAL MEMBRANES

1
DEVELOPMENT, ANATOMY, AND FUNCTION
OF THE SEROSAL MEMBRANES

DEVELOPMENT

The intraembryonic coelomic cavity appears at first as a number of isolated spaces within the lateral and cardiogenic mesoderms. These spaces coalesce to form a horseshoe-shaped cavity, the curve of which is the future pericardial cavity and the lateral parts of the future pleural and peritoneal cavities (14). The intraembryonic coelom divides the lateral mesoderm into somatic and splanchnic layers that form the linings of the primitive coelomic cavity. With continued development, the portion of the coelom that is intraembryonic is closed off ventrally from the extraembryonic part; the area around the umbilical cord is the last to close (fig. 1-1). During this process, the original right and left coelomic cavities advance toward each other and meet in the midline. The lateral halves of the pericardial cavity are the first part of the intraembryonic coelom formed by the splitting of the mesoderm and the first part completed by union of the cavities. In the midportion of the embryo, layers of splanchnic mesoderm couple to form the various mesenteries, and mesoderm ventral to the gut attenuates and the cavities coalesce.

The single coelomic space is partitioned into thoracic and abdominal portions by the formation of the septum transversum, the first part of the diaphragm to appear, and by pleuroperitoneal folds that arise from the body walls to join the septum. The pleural cavities are partitioned from the pericardial cavity by bilateral pleuropericardial folds, which also join the septum transversum (3).

The septum transversum originates in the cervical area of the embryo and moves caudad, so that by the second month of gestation it is at the level of the first lumbar vertebra. As it descends, it carries nerve fibers that form the phrenic nerves. The lungs also begin their development cephalically as buds from the endoderm projecting into the early pleuropericardial folds from the mesodermal ridge on each side (fig. 1-2) (3).

Separation of the pericardial and pleural cavities is completed first on the right side; a persistent communication between both cavities is usually present on the left (12). The diaphragm is derived from the septum transversum, forming the central tendon; the two pleuroperitoneal membranes; muscular portions from the dorsal and lateral body walls; and the mesentery of the esophagus.

The parietal membranes of pleura, peritoneum, and pericardium derive from somatic mesoderm; the visceral membranes derive from splanchnic mesoderm. The membranes are formed by a layer of persisting mesenchymal tissue with a flattened surface layer of cells which becomes the mesothelium. These layers appear to retain the potentiality to differentiate in a number of ways (12).

GROSS ANATOMY

The pleura is continuous over the surface of the pleural cavities and their contents. The visceral pleura covers the lungs, including the interlobar fissures. The parietal pleura lines the thoracic wall, the lateral aspect of the mediastinum, the suprapleural membrane, the thoracic inlet, and the thoracic surface of the diaphragm. The visceral pleura receives its blood supply from the bronchial arteries and the parietal pleura from the systemic circulation: the intercostal, internal mammary, and phrenic arteries. The venous return is parallel.

Both aspects of the pleura have an extensive lymphatic plexus. Lymphatics from visceral pleura drain to the pulmonary hilar lymph nodes, while those of the anterior parietal pleura pass into the intercostal network. Lymph flow from diaphragmatic pleura is to the lower mediastinal

1

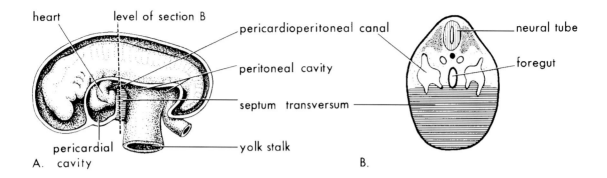

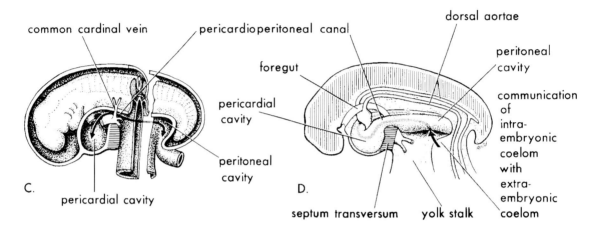

Figure 1-1
BODY CAVITIES AND MESENTERIES AT 24 DAYS' GESTATION

The drawing shows development and relationship of the pericardial cavity, pericardioperitoneal canals, septum transversum, and intraembryonic and extraembryonic coeloms.

A: The lateral wall of the pericardial cavity has been removed to show the heart.

B: Transverse section illustrating the relationship of the pericardioperitoneal canals to the septum transversum (partial diaphragm) and the foregut.

C: Lateral view with the heart removed. The embryo has been sectioned transversely to show the continuity of the intraembryonic and extraembryonic coeloms or body cavities.

D: Sketch showing the pericardioperitoneal canals arising from the dorsal wall of the pericardial cavity and passing on each side of the foregut to join the peritoneal cavity. The arrows show the communication of the extraembryonic coelom with the intraembryonic coelom and the continuity of the intraembryonic coelom. (Fig. 9-4 from Moore KL. The developing human. Clinically oriented embryology. 3d ed. Philadelphia: WB Saunders Co, 1982:167–78.)

lymph nodes. Drainage from the lower parietal pleura is to the retroperitoneal lymph nodes in the region of the adrenals and kidneys. There is also an outward flow of lymph from the lung parenchyma to the visceral pleura, assisted by valves in the lymphatics. This helps to explain spread of intrapulmonary tumor to the visceral pleura (13).

The vagus and sympathetic trunks innervate the visceral pleura and these are devoid of pain fibers. The parietal pleura is supplied with sensory nerve fibers from the intercostal nerves. The central portion of the diaphragm receives its innervation from the phrenic nerve and the rest from lower intercostal and abdominal wall nerves (8).

The peritoneal cavity is lined by a continuous serous membrane, except for the ostia of the Fallopian tubes. The visceral peritoneum covers the intra-abdominal organs and their mesenteries. The parietal peritoneum lines the abdominal wall, the pelvis, and the inferior surface of the diaphragm. It also covers part of the anterior surfaces of certain essentially retroperitoneal viscera (4). The peritoneal cavity has four main divisions: the supracolic, the right and left infracolic, and the pelvic. Due to

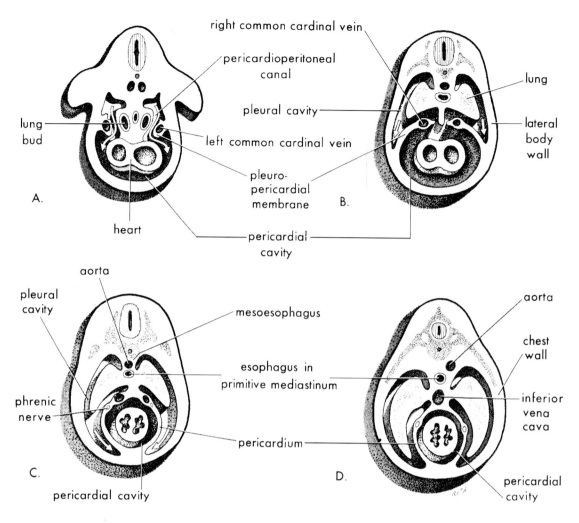

Figure 1-2
STAGES IN THE DEVELOPMENT OF THE PLEURAL CAVITIES

Schematic drawings of transverse section through an embryo cranial to the septum transversum, illustrating successive stages in the separation of the pleural cavities from the pericardial cavity. Growth and development of the lungs, expansion of the pleural cavities, and formation of the fibrous pericardium are also shown.

A: Five weeks. The arrows indicate the communications between the pericardioperitoneal canals and the pericardial cavity.

B: Six weeks. The arrows indicate development of the pleural cavities as extension of the pericardioperitoneal canals and expansion of the pleural cavities into the body wall.

C: Seven weeks. Expansion of the pleural cavities ventrally around the heart is shown. The pleuropericardial membranes are now fused in the midline with each other and with the mesoderm ventral to the esophagus.

D: Eight weeks. Continued expansion of the lungs and pleural cavities and formation of the fibrous pericardium and chest wall are illustrated. (Fig. 9-5 from Moore KL. The developing human. Clinically oriented embryology. 3rd ed. Philadelphia: WB Saunders, 1982:167–78.)

the obliquity of the small intestinal mesentery, the right infracolic space tapers inferiorly and the left tapers superiorly. These partitions affect the passage of fluid within the abdominal cavity (15).

The splanchnic arterial vessels supply most of the peritoneum and mesenteries and venous drainage is by splanchnic veins and the portal system. A limited portion obtains its blood supply from the lower intercostal and subcostal, lumbar, and iliac arteries. The peritoneal lymphatics follow the corresponding blood vessels. Efferent lymphatic vessels from the intestinal mucosa communicate with the intramuscular and subserosal plexus. After a short distance in the mesentery, these vessels unite to form collecting trunks and valves and the lymph passes through groups of lymph nodes and "milk spots" (lymphoid aggregates in the omentum). These efferent channels ultimately join to form an intestinal trunk which drains the part of bowel supplied by the superior mesenteric artery and empties into the cysterna chyli or the left lumbar trunk (9). Left and right lumbar lymphatic trunks carry lymph from the left side of the colon, the kidneys, adrenal glands, gonads, and lower extremities (10). Lymphatic vessels in the serosa on both sides of the diaphragm have extensive communications; those on the right are larger and convey more fluid than those on the left side.

The parietal and visceral layers have different innervations in the peritoneum and in the pleura. The former is innervated by the spinal nerves supplying the abdominal wall and these contain sensory pain fibers. The visceral peritoneum receives only sympathetic nerve fibers and is not pain sensitive.

The anatomic features of the pericardium and tunica vaginalis testis conform to the same anatomic principles as those of the pleura and peritoneum.

MICROSCOPIC ANATOMY

All serous membranes consist of a single layer of flat mesothelial cells resting on a basement membrane, with a submesothelial layer of connective tissue of variable thickness (fig. 1-3). The mesothelial cells range in diameter from 16 to 40 μm, have abundant cytoplasm, and have a centrally placed round nucleus, which may contain a small nucleolus.

There are differences in the histologic appearance of visceral and parietal pleurae. The microvilli of the visceral pleura tend to be more abundant than those of the parietal pleura. Gaps between parietal mesothelial cells that communicate with the underlying lymphatics are a feature seen only in the parietal pleura (17,18). Electron microscopy shows that the mesothelial cells have fairly dense cytoplasm that contains ribosomes, rough-surfaced endoplasmic reticulum, and a moderate number of mitochondria. There may be micropinocytotic vesicles in the cell membrane. Though junctional complexes and desmosomes are relatively abundant, they are discontinuous and diffusion of molecules between cells is feasible (7). One of the most prominent ultrastructural features of mesothelial cells is the presence of long and slender surface microvilli (figs. 1-4, 1-5). The microvilli measure

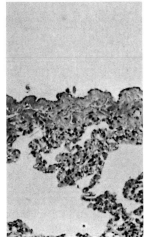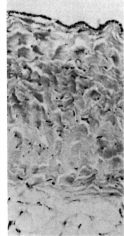

Figure 1-3
NORMAL SEROUS MEMBRANE
Left: Visceral pleura (X125).
Right: Parietal pericardium (X125). The submesothelial fibrous layer is much thicker in the parietal pericardium. (Hematoxylin and eosin stain) (Fig. 3 from Fascicle 20, 2nd series.)

up to 3.0 μm in length and 0.1 μm in diameter and are more abundant in the caudal portions of the pleura (6). The microvilli appear to be most abundant on the surfaces of tissues or organs that move about most actively (2,18), and it is believed that they serve to entrap mucosubstances that reduce friction at these sites.

Ultrastructurally, the mesothelial cells rest over a delicate basal layer. The underlying connective tissue contains variable amounts of collagen and elastic fibers, fibroblast-like cells, lymphatics, and capillaries. Ultrastructural studies of the diaphragmatic peritoneum have revealed gaps at points where mesothelial cells come in contact with the terminal lymphatics. At these points the mesothelial basal lamina is attenuated or missing, and the lymphatic endothelium lacks a basal lamina. Studies in animals have shown that pleural and peritoneal mesothelia have stomata allowing direct continuity between mesothelium and lymphatic endothelium (figs. 1-6, 1-7) (18).

FUNCTIONAL PROPERTIES

Under normal conditions there is a small amount of liquid between serosal surfaces. The mechanisms of pleural liquid and solute exchange have been recently reviewed (16). In addition to providing an almost frictionless lining

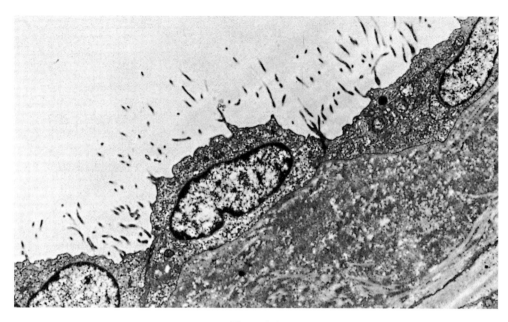

Figure 1-4
MESOTHELIAL CELL
Branching microvilli project from the surface of the flat mesothelial cells of human pleura (X6000). (Fig. 4 from Fascicle 20, 2nd series.)

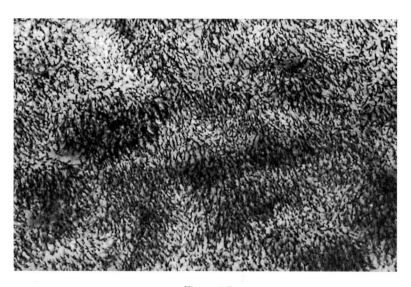

Figure 1-5
SURFACE OF MESOTHELIAL CELLS
In this scanning electron microscopic view of visceral rat pleura, the profusion of microvilli gives the surface a rough appearance (X5500). (Fig. 5 from Fascicle 20, 2nd series.)

to the spaces in which the various contractile and expansile viscera function, the serous membranes are continuously involved in fluid transport. The pleural space, i.e., the distance separating the visceral and parietal pleura, is 5 to 10 μm wide and occupied by fluid and free cells. The fluid contains glycosaminoglycans, particularly hyaluronate, which act as lubricants.

Hydrostatic and colloidal osmotic pressures in the serosal capillaries move fluid from the blood stream to the pleural space and in the reverse direction. The greater hydrostatic pressure in the

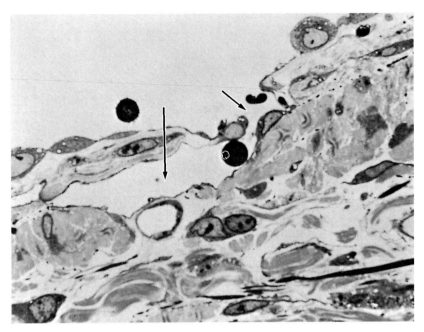

Figure 1-6
STOMA ON MESOTHELIAL SURFACE
A lymphatic lacuna (long arrow) opens onto the mesothelial surface via a narrow stoma (short arrow). The diameters of two round mononuclear cells are larger than the narrowest portion of the stoma (X1000). (1-μm thick epon section). (Fig. 9 from Wang NS. The preformed stomas connecting the pleural cavity and the lymphatics in the parietal pleura. Am Rev Respir Dis 1975;111:12–20.)

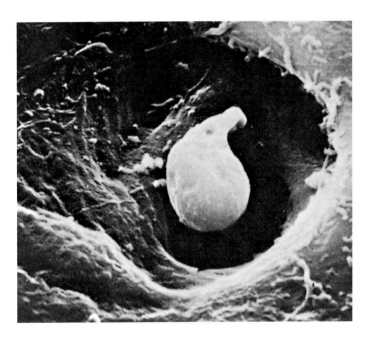

Figure 1-7
STOMA ON MESOTHELIAL SURFACE
Stoma on the subcostal parietal pleura of a rabbit. There is a deformed red blood cell in the opening (X5500). (Fig. 1 from Wang NS. The preformed stomas connecting the pleural cavity and the lymphatics in the parietal pleura. Am Rev Respir Dis 1975;111:12–20.)

systemic circulation of the parietal pleura than the pulmonary circulation favors a transudation of fluid from the arterial ends of the capillaries of that layer into the pleural space, with reabsorption into the venous ends of the capillaries of the visceral pleura (5). The visceral pleura is more highly vascularized than the parietal pleura.

About 10 to 20 percent of pleural fluid passes into the lymphatics of the parietal pleura. Larger molecules, particularly proteins, enter directly into lymphatics. Particulate matter and cells are also taken up by lymphatics, principally in the lower mediastinal and costal areas in animals (1,5,16), but not by the visceral pleura. Particulate matter in the peritoneal cavity passes through the lymphatics of the diaphragm. Respiratory muscular activity is known to affect the flow of lymph.

Obstruction of the lymphatic channels or lymph nodes may cause or increase serous effu-sion. Particulate matter, fibrosis, or neoplasm can effectively block lymph flow through nodes. The retained fluid, with its raised protein content, aggravates the effusion. Thickening of the pleura of the chest wall may prevent absorption of fluid by sealing lymphatics. Since ascitic fluid drains through the diaphragm into the pleural cavities, particularly the right, an overload of the lymphatic drainage system may result in retention of fluid in the thorax.

There has been much investigation of fluid transport via the mesothelial cell. While fluid transmission by micropinocytotic vesicles has been suggested, diffuse intracellular passage of fluid and particles has also been demonstrated. Equalization of protein and salt composition of the serous fluid has been ascribed to pinocytosis (11). Other studies indicate that the intercellular clefts are the major sites of fluid and solute transport across the peritoneal membrane (7).

REFERENCES

1. Albertine KH, Wiener-Kronish P, Staub NC. The structure of the parietal pleura and its relationship to pleural liquid dynamics in sheep. Anat Rec 1984;208:401–9.
2. Andrews PM, Porter KR. The ultrastructural morphology and possible functional significance of mesothelial microvilli. Anat Rec 1973;177:409–26.
3. Arey LB. Developmental anatomy. A textbook and laboratory manual of embryology. 7th ed. Philadelphia: W.B. Saunders Co, 1965:284–93.
4. Bender MD, Ockner RK. Diseases of the peritoneum, mesentery, and diaphragm. In: Sleisenger MH, Fordtran JS, eds. Gastrointestinal disease. 2nd ed. Philadelphia: W.B. Saunders Co, 1978:1947–8.
5. Black LF. The pleural space and pleural fluid. Mayo Clin Proc 1972;47:493–506.
6. Carter D, True L, Otis C. Serous membranes. In: Sternberg SS, ed. Histology for pathologists. New York: Raven Press, 1992:499–514.
7. Cotran RS, Karnovsky MJ. Ultrastructural studies on the permeability of the mesothelium to horseradish peroxidase. J Cell Biol 1968;37:123–37.
8. Green RA, Johnston RF. Introduction to pleural disease. In: Baum GL, ed. Textbook of pulmonary diseases. 2nd ed. Boston: Little, Brown and Co, 1974:941–57.
9. Haagensen CD. General anatomy of the lymphatic system. In: Haagensen CD, ed. The lymphatics in cancer. Philadelphia: W.B. Saunders Co, 1972:22–41.
10. Hollingshead WH. Textbook of anatomy. 3rd ed. Hagerstown: Harper and Row, 1974:640.
11. Ivanova VF. Role of the mesothelium of the parietal peritoneum in the process of absorption of true solutions and India ink suspension from the abdominal cavity. Bull Exp Biol Med 1976;82:1258–61.
12. Langman J. Coelomic cavity and mesenteries. In: 3rd ed. Baltimore: Williams & Wilkins, 1975:303–17.
13. Lowell JR. Anatomy and physiology. In: Pleural effusions. A comprehensive review. Baltimore: University Park Press, 1977:7–11.
14. Moore KL. Coelomic cavity and mesenteries. In: Moore KL, ed. The developing human. Clinically oriented embryology. Philadelphia: W.B. Saunders Co, 1982:303–17.
15. Morson BC. The peritoneum. In: Symmers WS, ed. Systemic pathology. 2nd ed. London: Churchill Livingston, 1978:1179–97.
16. Pistolesi M, Minati M, Giuntini C. Pleural liquid and solute exchange. Am Rev Respir Dis 1989;140:825–47.
17. Wang N. The preformed stomas connecting the pleural cavity and the lymphatics in the parietal pleura. Am Rev Respir Dis 1975;111:12–20.
18. _____. The regional differences of pleural mesothelial cells in rabbits. Am Rev Respir Dis 1974;110:623–33.

2

REACTIVE PROCESSES IN THE SEROSAL MEMBRANES

INJURY AND REGENERATION

Experimental studies have permitted detailed observation of the effects of injury on serous membranes. Within a few hours, a denuded or injured serous surface is covered by a deposit of fibrin, polymorphonuclear leukocytes, and mononuclear cells identified as macrophages (8,9,15, 16,19). After one day, macrophages predominate on the surface. By the second and third days, the surface cells start to show evidence of flattening (19,21). If the injury is more than superficial, mesenchymal cells resembling fibroblasts also appear at this stage (8,16). By the fifth to eighth day, there is a continuous surface layer of flattened cells similar or identical in their light microscopic and ultrastructural characteristics to normal mesothelium (8,19,21), and a basal lamina has formed. Underlying granulation tissue becomes less vascular and the fibroblasts align themselves parallel to the surface. After several weeks, repair is essentially complete.

The mechanisms of surface mesothelium renewal are controversial. Some have found evidence that the mesothelium is formed by macrophages deposited on the denuded surface (9,19, 21); others have proposed that desquamated mesothelial cells reattach to denuded surfaces (16,23,24). Most observers have found no evidence that ingrowth of mesothelial cells from the margins of the denuded area is significantly involved in the repair process. However, substantial mesothelial ingrowth over an injured serosal surface has been observed (24). Based on experimental light and electron microscopic studies of the healing of peritoneal mesothelium, Raftery (16) proposed that new mesothelium develops from subperitoneal perivascular connective cells; it is unclear whether these are primitive mesenchymal cells or fibroblasts. Recent evidence, based on immunohistochemical studies with monoclonal antibodies to intermediate filaments, shows that these subserosal mesenchymal cells have unique properties, which distinguish them from fibroblasts elsewhere in the body (fig. 2-1). Normal surface mesothelium expresses low and high molecular weight cytokeratins while the underlying, fibroblast-like submesothelial cells express only vimentin when at rest; when proliferating, these submesothelial cells coexpress low molecular weight cytokeratins as well (1). Thus, rather than fibroblasts, these cells may be regarded as multipotential mesenchymal cells. When surface differentiation occurs, these cells add high molecular weight cytokeratins to their intermediate filament phenotype, and vimentin production is shut off (2). Additionally, in common with proliferating fibroblasts, the cells switch on the production of contractile proteins such as actin, in concert with their migratory capacity (1). The earlier observations of Raftery suggesting that mesothelia regenerate from subserosal cells has gained strong support from these immunohistochemical observations and the diagnostic usefulness of the intermediate filament phenotype exhibited by the various subtypes of mesothelioma is shown. Nonetheless, the existence of a multipotential or mesothelial stem cell is still debatable. Whitaker et al. (22) believe that the desquamated surface mesothelial cell is the main cell responsible for restoration of the surface mesothelium: irradiation of rat testis prevented mesothelial healing, whereas irradiation followed by serosal lavages containing mesothelial cells from other injured animals allowed healing to proceed. These experiments support the view that remesothelialization derives from free-floating mesothelial cells. The subserosal, keratin-positive spindle cells may, according to these authors, be involved in serosal repair but are unlikely to be responsible for the repopulation of the surface mesothelium.

HYPERPLASIA

Hyperplasia, shedding of mesothelium, and fibrosis are common reactions to persistent serosal injury and frequently cause diagnostic problems in the evaluation of fluids and biopsies from the serous cavities. It is difficult to differentiate mesothelial hyperplasia from epithelial-type mesothelioma and scar tissue from fibrous or desmoplastic mesothelioma, especially if tissue

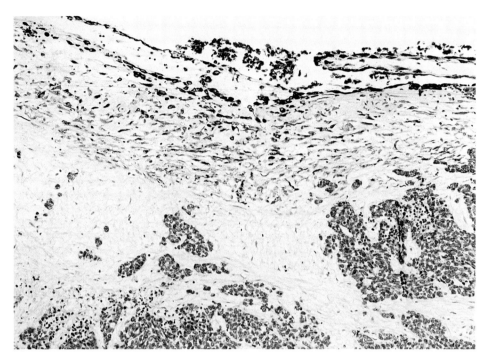

Figure 2-1
REGENERATING MESOTHELIAL CELLS
Regenerating mesothelial cells at the site of a metastasis of undifferentiated carcinoma to the peritoneum that were stained with a cocktail of monoclonal antibodies to keratins of low molecular weight. Note the layer of keratin-positive spindle cells sharply demarcated from the underlying mesenchyme. The more superficial cells have abundant cytoplasm and have acquired epithelial features.

available for study is small or derived from only one or two biopsy sites.

There is considerable overlap between the histologic characteristics of mesothelial hyperplasia and well-differentiated epithelial mesothelioma (3,14). Hyperplastic mesothelial cells may form a thin layer (figs. 2-2, 2-3) or solid nodules (fig. 2-4). They may extend a short distance into the underlying tissue and thus simulate neoplastic invasion (figs. 2-4, 2-5). Occasionally, they align in a tubular or trabecular pattern or form papillae (fig. 2-6). The nodular form of mesothelial hyperplasia is not uncommon in hernial sacs (18). In cytologic preparations, hyperplastic mesothelial cells may show many changes: enlargement, variation in size, increased optical density of cytoplasm, cytoplasmic vacuolation, increased nuclear-cytoplasmic ratio, nuclear chromatin irregularities, and pseudoglandular clustering (fig. 2-7). Binucleation is sometimes seen and occasional mitoses may be noted. These cytologic abnormalities may also be predominant in effusions accompa-

nying well-differentiated mesotheliomas, but in such cases the degree of hyperplasia and the presence of at least a small number of poorly differentiated mesothelial cells usually indicate the neoplastic nature of the process. Clumps or morulae of cells, especially when plentiful, also favor tumor over hyperplasia. Large sheets of mesothelial cells without stromal support may be seen in cell blocks and biopsies and can be misinterpreted as neoplastic.

It is appropriate to use the term *atypical mesothelial hyperplasia* for cases in which proliferating mesothelium shows some, but not all, of the cytologic or histologic characteristics of well-differentiated mesothelioma.

Histologic appearances identical to those of mesothelial hyperplasia may occur in parts of diffuse mesotheliomas of epithelial character or on the serous surfaces adjacent to any type of tumor involving mesothelium. In small biopsies, these characteristics sometimes predominate. The degree of cellular proliferation and atypia is important in making a distinction between hyperplasia

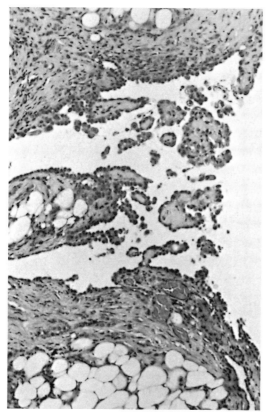

Figure 2-2
MESOTHELIAL HYPERPLASIA

Papillary hyperplasia is seen on a peritoneal surface. Swollen mesothelial cells cover the papillary projections. There is also a superficial zone of fibrosis (X125). (Fig. 9 from Fascicle 20, 2nd Series.)

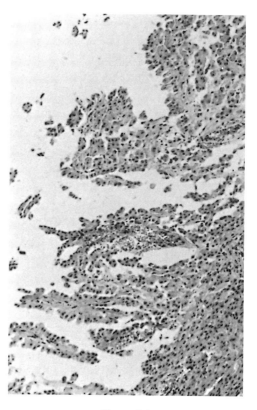

Figure 2-3
MESOTHELIAL HYPERPLASIA

Papillary and solid mesothelial cell proliferation is seen in this biopsy of one of a number of small nodules on the mesentery. The patient was well 4 years later (X125). (Fig. 1 from Foyle A, Al-Jabi M, McCaughey WT. Papillary peritoneal tumors in women. Am J Surg Pathol 1981;5:241–9.)

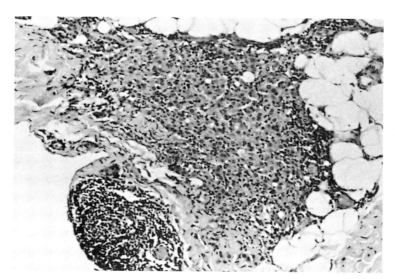

Figure 2-4
MESOTHELIAL HYPERPLASIA

A nodule of hyperplastic mesothelium is just beneath the inner surface of a hernia sac. There is also some lymphocytic infiltration (X125). (Fig. 12 from Fascicle 20, 2nd Series.)

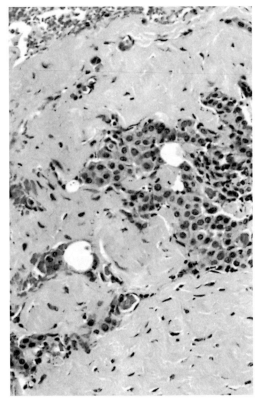

Figure 2-5
MESOTHELIAL INFILTRATION

The wall of an umbilical hernia sac showed numerous foci of mesothelial infiltration similar to that seen here. The patient was well 1 year later. An earlier repair of the hernia sac 6 years previously had also shown mesothelial hyperplasia (X125). (Fig. 13 from Fascicle 20, 2nd Series.)

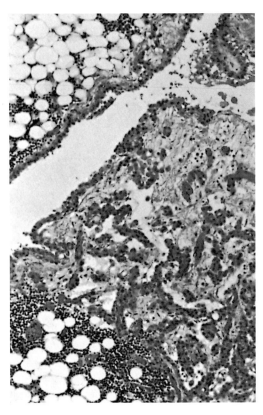

Figure 2-6
MESOTHELIAL INFILTRATION

Cords of mesothelial cells extend deep to the surface of the omentum. The patient had multiple peritoneal granulations at laparotomy. Ascites was still present 6 years later (X125). (Fig. 2 from Foyle A, Al-Jabi M, McCaughey WT. Papillary peritoneal tumors in women. Am J Surg Pathol 1981;5:241–9.)

Figure 2-7
CYTOLOGY OF HYPERPLASTIC
MESOTHELIUM

A group of mesothelial cells was found in a pleural effusion of cardiac origin. The nuclei show some irregularity and occasional cells are binucleate. There is some vacuolation of the deeply staining cytoplasm (X160). (Plate IA from Fascicle 20, 2nd Series.)

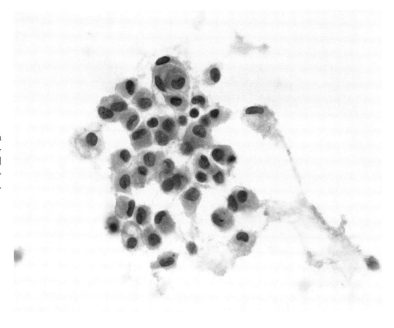

and neoplasia in these cases. Necrosis of hyperplastic-appearing mesothelium is strongly suggestive of mesothelioma (14). Knowledge of any antecedent irritative process, such as pneumonia, infarction, or pneumothorax, in an underlying viscus or radiologic or visual evidence of tumor may help with the evaluation. Informed assessment of the cytologic preparation from an associated effusion is often particularly useful, because it is more likely to give a representative sample of the proliferating mesothelium in a large cavity than a small biopsy specimen. A small number of slowly growing mesotheliomas begin with what initially looks like mesothelial hyperplasia (4,10). We have seen this phenomenon ourselves, with the hyperplasia occasionally developing years before the mesothelioma. Recent reports suggest that mutation of the p53 tumor suppressor gene may be present in a high proportion of mesotheliomas but not in hyperplastic mesothelium, and that immunostaining for p53 protein may be of diagnostic value (6,11,13,17).

Injury of various types, as well as the presence of nearby neoplasms, often results in a reactive proliferation of elongated cells of fibroblastic appearance immediately below the serous membrane. Nuclear irregularity or hyperchromasia in these cells may resemble a tumor. Additionally, cells resembling the strap cells of rhabdomyosarcoma have been described in such reactive hyperplasia (18). Distinction of these reactive processes from sarcoma and sarcomatous mesotheliomas are discussed in chapter 4.

Fibrosis of the serous membranes, especially the pleura, is quite common and is usually the end result of inflammatory or irritative processes. We have often seen cases of pleural fibrosis diagnosed as desmoplastic mesothelioma of fibrous pleurisy, but in which follow-up showed no evidence of progression or any causative process.

Small lesions, apparently composed of hyperplastic mesothelium resembling histiocytoid hemangioma, were recently noted in the heart and pericardium (12). These lesions were found at the time of cardiac surgery and were believed to represent a form of nodular mesothelial hyperplasia, possibly as a reactive process in response to previous cardiac catheterization. The lesions are characterized by an admixture of histiocytes and strips and tubular arrays of me-

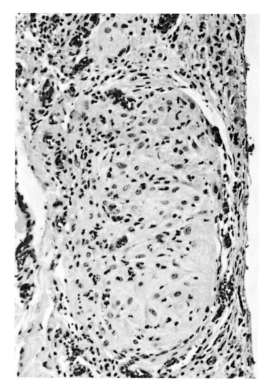

Figure 2-8
DECIDUAL REACTION IN PERITONEUM
There is a nodule of plump decidual cells just beneath the surface (X125). (Fig. 15 from Fascicle 20, 2nd Series.)

sothelial cells. The term *mesothelial/monocytic incidental cardiac excrescences (MICE)* has been suggested for these lesions (20). More recently it has been suggested that these "lesions" may represent an artifact produced during cardiac surgery by the cardiotomy suction with resulting accumulation and compaction of aspirated mesothelial surface cells (5).

METAPLASIA

Squamous metaplasia of mesothelium has occasionally been noted (7). Endometriosis and endosalpingiosis, and the proliferative epithelial peritoneal lesions associated with some ovarian serous tumors of low malignant potential, are thought by many to represent metaplasia of mesothelium (chapter 5). The decidual reaction of pregnancy (fig. 2-8) and the rare condition known as leiomyomatosis peritonealis disseminata are examples of metaplasia occurring in the submesothelial layers of the peritoneum.

REFERENCES

1. Bolen JW, Hammar SP, McNutt MA. Reactive and neoplastic serosal tissue. A light-microscopic, ultrastructural, and immunocytochemical study. Am J Surg Pathol 1986;10:34–47.

2. _____, Hammar SP, McNutt MA. Serosal tissue: reactive tissue as a model for understanding mesotheliomas. Ultrastruct Pathol 1987;11:251–62.

3. Carter D, True L, Otis CN. Serous membranes. In: Sternberg SS, ed. Histology for pathologists. New York: Raven Press, 1992:499–514.

4. Churg J. Peritoneal mesothelioma. Environ Health Perspect 1974;9:317–8.

5. Courtice RW, Stinson WA, Walley VM. Tissue fragments recovered at cardiac surgery masquerading as tumoral proliferations. Evidence suggesting iatrogenic or artefactual origin and common occurrence. Am J Surg Pathol 1994;18:167–74.

6. Côté RJ, Jhanwar SC, Novick S, Pellicer A. Genetic alterations of the p53 gene are a feature of malignant mesotheliomas. Cancer Res 1991;51:5410–6.

7. Crome L. Squamous metaplasia of the peritoneum. J Pathol Bacteriol 1950;62:61–8.

8. Ellis H, Harrison W, Hugh TB. The healing of peritoneum under normal and pathological conditions. Br J Surg 1965;52:471–6.

9. Eskeland G. Regeneration of parietal peritoneum in rats. 1. A light microscopical study. Acta Pathol Microbiol Scand [B] 1966;68:355–78.

10. Hellström P, Friman C, Teppo L. Malignant mesothelioma of 17 years' duration with high pleural fluid concentrate of hyaluronate. Scand J Resp Dis 1977; 58:97–102.

11. Kafiri G, Thomas DM, Shepherd NA, Krausz T, Lane DP, Hall PA. p53 expression is common in malignant mesothelioma. Histopathology 1992;21:331–4.

12. Luthringer DJ, Virmani R, Weiss SW, Rosai J. A distinctive cardiovascular lesion resembling histiocytoid (epithelioid) hemangioma: evidence suggesting mesothelial participation. Am J Surg Pathol 1990;14:993–1000.

13. Mayall FG, Goddard H, Gibbs AR. p53 immunostaining in the distinction between benign and malignant mesothelial proliferations using formalin-fixed paraffin sections. J Pathol 1992;168:377–81.

14. McCaughey WT, Al-Jabi M. Differentiation of serosal hyperplasia and neoplasia in biopsies. Pathol Ann 1986;21 (Pt 1):271–93.

15. Moalli PA, MacDonald JL, Goodglick LA, Kane AB. Acute injury and regeneration of the mesothelium in response to asbestos fibers. Am J Pathol 1987;128:426–45.

16. Raftery AT. Regeneration of parietal and visceral peritoneum in the immature animal: a light and electron microscopical study. Br J Surg 1973;60:969–75.

17. Ramael M, Lemmens G, Eerdekens C, et al. Immunoreactivity for p53 protein in malignant mesothelioma and non-neoplastic mesothelium. J Pathol 1992; 168:371–5.

18. Rosai J, Dehner LP. Nodular mesothelial hyperplasia in hernia sacs: a benign reactive condition simulating a neoplastic process. Cancer 1975;35:165–75.

19. Ryan GB, Grobty J, Majno G. Mesothelial injury and recovery. Am J Pathol 1973;71:93–112.

20. Veinot JP, Tazelaar HD, Edwards WD, Colby TV. Mesothelial/monocytic incidental cardiac excrescences: cardiac MICE. Modern Pathol 1994;7:9–16.

21. Watters WB, Buck RC. Scanning electron microscopy of mesothelial regeneration in the rat. Lab Invest 1972;26:604–9.

22. Whitaker D, Manning LS, Robinson DW, Shilkin KB. The pathobiology of mesothelium. In: Henderson DW, Shilkin KB, Langlois SL, Whitaker D, eds. Malignant mesothelioma. New York: Hemisphere Publishing, 1992:25–56.

23. _____, Papadimitriou J. Mesothelial healing: morphological and kinetic investigations. J Pathol 1985;145:159–75.

24. _____, Papadimitriou JM, Walters MN. The mesothelium and its reactions: a review. Crit Rev Toxicol 1982;10:81–144.

❖ ❖ ❖

3

PRIMARY TUMORS OF THE SEROSAL MEMBRANES

Tumors of the serous membranes were described with increasing frequency throughout the nineteenth century, amid growing controversy concerning their origin. Those who believed these tumors to be primary debated their histogenesis and, especially, the role of the serosal lining cells (mesothelium). Skepticism concerning the form of the primary serosal tumor, which subsequently became known as diffuse malignant mesothelioma (DMM), persisted well into the middle third of the present century, since some felt that many putative cancers of this type did not originate in serous membranes (8,11). This belief also fostered, for a time, the view that a definite diagnosis of DMM could only be made at autopsy and that even then an occult extraserosal primary tumor might easily have been missed.

In the second half of the nineteenth century, malignant tumors resembling DMM were often described by such designations as endothelioma, endothelial cancer, pleural cancer, and pleural sarcoma (8), but the details reported do not permit accurate classification of these neoplasms based on current knowledge and criteria. The first recorded use of the term mesothelium was by Minot in 1890; Adami used the term mesothelioma in 1909 (10).

Widespread acceptance of the existence of DMM as an entity grew out of a number of detailed pathologic studies from 1930 to 1960 (2,4,5,7). These studies brought about an increasing realization that diagnosis should be based on more positive considerations than exclusion of other sources of tumor at autopsy. The tumor was recognized to have distinctive gross characteristics and behavior, and a diversified microscopic structure that was at times highly specific. Support developed for the concept that mesothelium could produce tumors with either epithelial or mesenchymal characteristics, or both, and that this capacity was related to the mesodermal origin of the cell. Evidence supporting this belief was shown by Klemperer and Rabin in 1931 (5). These authors also divided primary pleural tumors into diffuse and localized forms, and expressed the opinion that diffuse tumors arose from mesothelium and localized tumors of a fibrous or mesenchymal nature originated from submesothelial areolar tissue. These localized fibrous tumors were subsequently thought to be of mesothelial origin by others and designated localized (or solitary) mesotheliomas. In the past decade, however, ultrastructural and immunohistochemical studies have shown that these tumors develop from submesothelial connective tissue. The division of pleural tumors into diffuse and localized types has been widely accepted by pathologists and clinicians for many years: localized tumors are usually fibrous and benign and diffuse tumors often appear epithelial, at least in part, and are nearly always malignant.

The arcane tumor now known as diffuse malignant mesothelioma would probably never have stimulated the interest of more than a small number of anatomic pathologists and oncologists were it not for the revelation by Wagner et al. in 1960 (9) that many persons with mesothelioma in South Africa had been exposed to asbestos. The etiologic relationship with asbestos was confirmed in the next decade in most western industrial countries and it became imperative, particularly for epidemiologic reasons, to identify DMM as accurately as possible; objective diagnosis, then as now, was heavily dependent on the pathology laboratory. It is now recognized that therapeutic radiation causes occasional cases of DMM (3); also the nonasbestiform zeolite fiber known as erionite has caused epidemics of DMM in certain remote areas of Turkey (1).

After 1950, increasing cases of DMM of pleura and peritoneum were recognized, as well as occasional cases arising from pericardium and tunica vaginalis testis. The spectrum of mesothelial neoplasms in the peritoneum of women is wider than in men, although DMM is much less common in the female peritoneum (6).

MESOTHELIOMA

Mesothelioma is a tumor derived from the lining cells (mesothelium) of a serous cavity. The tumor may be restricted to a small area of the

Table 3-1

CLASSIFICATION OF PRIMARY TUMORS OF SEROUS MEMBRANES

Localized
Mesothelial
    Adenomatoid tumor
    Benign cystic mesothelioma (multilocular
        peritoneal inclusion cyst) - some cases
    Mesothelial cyst, paratesticular region
Submesothelial
    Submesothelial fibroma (localized fibrous
        mesothelioma)
    Fibrosarcoma (malignant submesothelial
        fibrous tumor)
    Angioma, angiosarcoma
    Other soft tissue tumors

Diffuse
Mesothelial
    Malignant mesothelioma
        Epithelial
            Tubulopapillary
            Nonglandular (solid)
        Sarcomatous
        Biphasic
        Undifferentiated (poorly differentiated)
    Serous papillary carcinoma of peritoneum
    Borderline malignant serous papillary
        carcinoma of peritoneum
    Well-differentiated papillary mesothelioma of
        peritoneum
    Cystic malignant mesothelioma
Submesothelial
    Angiosarcoma
    Epithelioid hemangioendothelioma

affected membrane or involve the membrane multifocally or in a continuous manner. Tumors confined to a single area often have an adenomatoid or well-differentiated papillary structure, and are usually benign. They may also represent the early stages of DMM. Localized fibrous tumors of serous membrane appear to arise from submesothelial tissue. They are usually benign and should be called *submesothelial fibromas*. When malignant they are appropriately described as *submesothelial fibrosarcoma*. The main diffuse mesothelial tumor is *diffuse malignant mesothelioma (DMM)*. This is an aggressive neoplasm which characteristically involves serous membranes multifocally at an early stage and in its late stages encases the viscera in the affected body cavity. Microscopically, it may show epithelial or sarcomatous characteristics or be biphasic. Indolent forms of DMM occasionally occur and are usually of well-differentiated papillary or cystic character. Though serous papillary tumors arise from the surface epithelium (mesothelium) of the ovary or its extension into the ovary, these tumors and similar neoplasms of extraovarian peritoneal origin are not usually categorized as mesotheliomas.

CLASSIFICATION

A classification of primary serosal tumors, based on current views of their histogenesis, is seen in Table 3-1.

REFERENCES

1. Baris YI, Artvinli M, Sahin AA. Environmental mesothelioma in Turkey. Ann NY Acad Sci 1979;330:423–32.
2. Campbell WN. Pleural mesothelioma. Am J Pathol 1950;26:473–87.
3. Gilks B, Hegedus C, Freeman H, Fratkin L, Churg A. Malignant peritoneal mesothelioma after remote abdominal irradiation. Cancer 1988;61:2019–21.
4. Godwin MC. Diffuse mesotheliomas. With comment on their relation to localized fibrous mesotheliomas. Cancer 1957;10:298–319.
5. Klemperer P, Rabin CB. Primary neoplasms of the pleura. A report of five cases. Arch Pathol 1931;11:385–412.
6. McCaughey WT. Papillary peritoneal neoplasms in females. Pathol Ann 1985;(Pt 2):387–404.
7. _____. Primary tumors of the pleura. J Pathol Bacteriol 1958;76:517–29.
8. Robertson HE. Endothelioma of the pleura. J Cancer Res 1924;8:317–75.
9. Wagner JC, Sleggs CA, Marchand P. Diffuse pleural mesothelioma and asbestos exposure in the North Western Cape province. Brit J Industr Med 1960;17:260–71.
10. Whitaker D, Manning LS, Robinson DW, Shilkin KB. The pathobiology of mesothelium. In: Henderson DW, Shilkin KB, Langlois SL, Whitaker D, eds. Malignant mesothelioma. New York: Hemisphere Publishing 1992:25–56.
11. Willis RA. Pathology of tumours. 4th ed. London: Butterworths, 1967.

4
DIFFUSE MALIGNANT MESOTHELIOMA

Histogenesis. The mesothelial origin of primary diffuse malignant tumors of serous membranes is supported by the close resemblance between the effusion cytology and biopsy characteristics of tumor cells and hyperplastic mesothelium in diffuse tumors of epithelial form. Tissue culture studies (259,286) and electron microscopy (32,291) further support a mesothelial origin for mesothelioma. That neoplastic mesothelium has the capacity to diversify in other directions, and in particular, to form diffuse tumors of sarcomatous appearance, is supported by the existence of biphasic histologic forms of diffuse tumor in which sarcomatoid and epithelial tumor cell elements are admixed, and by the similar gross and behavioral characteristics of pure epithelial and pure sarcomatoid forms of diffuse tumor. There may be a multipotential subserosal cell capable of evolving into mesothelium or areolar tissue which accounts for the diverse histologic differentiation exhibited by mesotheliomas (31,328). The identification of mesothelium with embryonal mesoderm has led to the suggestion that the term *mesodermoma* be used to identify primary tumors of serous membranes (93).

Etiology and Pathogenesis. Although there were occasional previous references to serous membrane tumors in persons exposed to asbestos (33,181,325), Wagner and associates (312) gave the first epidemiologically significant evidence of a link between asbestos and mesotheliomas in 1960. In the following years, other studies confirmed this relationship on the basis of exposure histories (198,262), the finding of asbestos bodies in the lung (198), and the capacity of various types of asbestos to produce mesotheliomas when injected into the serosal cavities of experimental animals (277,310). An association between asbestos exposure and diffuse peritoneal mesothelioma was also established at that time (164,262). Recent evidence links asbestos exposure and the rare mesotheliomas arising in the pericardium (22,151) and the tunica vaginalis testis (52). Pericardial mesothelioma in man has also followed direct application of asbestos and fiberglass to pericardial membrane (61). Although mesothe-

lioma has yielded little to therapeutic assault, accurate diagnosis of the neoplasm continues to be essential because of its unique role in assessing the carcinogenic effects of asbestos.

Experimental studies suggest that the carcinogenicity of asbestos in serous membranes is related particularly to its fibrous structure (282,303) and that differences in the dimensions of the various types of asbestos fiber (fig. 4-1) explain variations in their carcinogenicity (303). Fibers less than 0.25 μm in diameter and greater than 8 μm in length are more potent than shorter, thicker forms (282). Erionite, a fibrous form of zeolite not related to asbestos but with similar physical properties, has been implicated in outbreaks of diffuse malignant mesothelioma (DMM) in Turkey (15,16), suggesting that any nonasbestos mineral fiber may cause DMM if its physical characteristics are similar to those of asbestos. This is further supported by the observation that DMM can be produced experimentally by a variety of nonasbestiform mineral fibers (281), including erionite (292). So far, there is no evidence of an excess of DMM among employees of the large man-made mineral fiber industry which exists in a number of countries although there may be an excess of lung cancer with some types of exposure (338). The chemical composition of the six types of asbestos fiber is shown in Table 4-1. Chrysotile is a serpentine mineral; the others are all amphiboles. Chrysotile accounted for 95 percent of the asbestos used commercially in the past.

There is no evidence that the chemical composition of asbestos fibers is related to their carcinogenicity. However, the carcinogenicity may be effected by direct and indirect mechanisms: directly by the physical interaction of fibers with target cells and indirectly by the production of chemical mediators by inflammatory cells attracted to the area where asbestos is deposited (314).

Chrysotile, amosite, and crocidolite, the forms of asbestos that have been of greatest commercial importance, have all been etiologically linked to DMM, as has the tremolite form of asbestos, a frequent contaminant of chrysotile

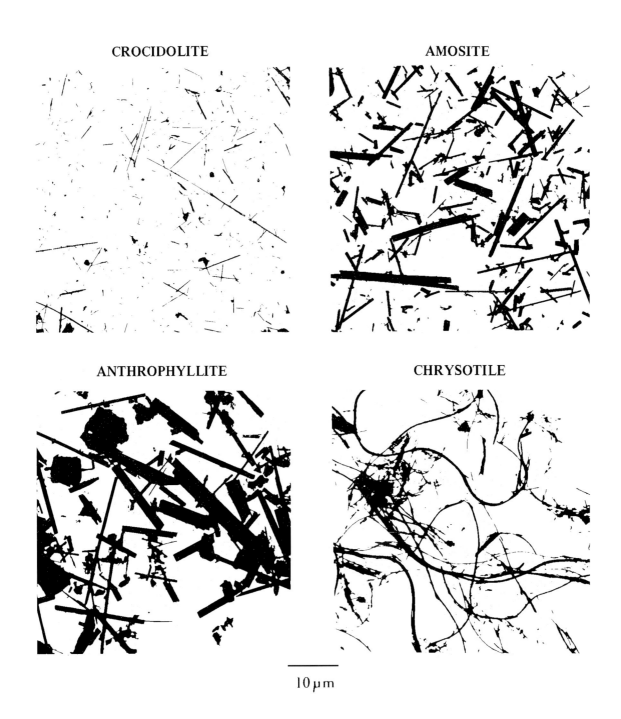

CROCIDOLITE

AMOSITE

ANTHROPHYLLITE

CHRYSOTILE

10 µm

Figure 4-1
ASBESTOS FIBERS

Transmission electron micrographs of powdered asbestos minerals, illustrating the main types of fibers at the same magnification. Note the rectilinear shape of the amphibole fiber (crocidolite, amosite, anthrophyllite) compared with the curved and twisted morphology of chrysotile fiber, and the different diameters of the fibers (X1700). (Fig. 1 from Timbrell V. Physical factors as etiological mechanisms. In: Bogovski P, Gilson JG, Timbrell V, Wagner JC, eds. Biological effects of asbestos. Lyon: International Agency for Research on Cancer, 1973:295–303.)

Table 4-1

CHEMICAL COMPOSITION OF ASBESTIFORM MINERALS*

Asbestos Variety	Chemical Formula
Chrysotile	$Mg_3 Si_2 O_5 (OH)_4$
Crocidolite	$Na_2 Fe_3{+}{+} Fe_2{+}{+}{+} Si_8 O_{22} (OH)_2$
Amosite	$(Fe\text{-}Mg)_7 Si_8 O_{22} (OH)_2 \quad Fe > 5$
Tremolite	$Ca_2 Mg_5 Si_8 O_{22} (OH)_2$
Anthophyllite	$(Mg\text{-}Fe)_7 Si_8 O_{22} (OH)_2 \quad Mg > 6$
Actinolite	$Ca_2 Mg Fe_5 Si_8 O_{22} (OH)_2$

*From reference 250a.

ore. The risk of developing DMM is greatest with crocidolite exposure and least with chrysotile exposure (132). However, amosite is more frequently associated with DMM in North America than is crocidolite (Table 4-2) (203).

Table 4-2 summarizes the numbers and types of asbestos fibers found in the lungs of 99 (76 male, 23 female) North American patients with DMM. Five mineral types of asbestos (chrysotile, amosite, crocidolite, tremolite, anthophyllite) were found in the lung specimens. In the case of amosite, 26 male patients had more than 1×10^6 fibers/g of dried lung tissue as compared with 8 controls; for crocidolite, 15 male patients had more than 1×10^6 fibers compared with 5 controls. Of the 76 males, 86 percent had more than 1×10^6 chrysotile fibers/g of dried lung, but there was no difference in the chrysotile fiber content between patients and their paired controls. Six male patients

Table 4-2

ASBESTOS IN THE LUNGS OF PATIENTS WITH DIFFUSE MALIGNANT MESOTHELIOMA*

Number of Fibers	Chrysotile Cases	Chrysotile Control	Amosite Cases	Amosite Control	Crocidolite Cases	Crocidolite Control	Anthophyllite Cases	Anthophyllite Control	Tremolite Cases	Tremolite Control
Males										
None	3	1	37	47	47	60	58	61	29	31
Less than 1	8	11	13	21	14	11	11	12	33	38
1 to 10	38	38	14	7	6	5	4	3	10	16
10 to 100	25	22	8	1	8	—	2	—	3	1
100 to 1000	2	2	3	—	1	—	—	—	—	—
1000 and over	—	2	1	—	—	—	—	—	1	—
Females										
None	—	—	17	15	15	16	18	17	7	9
Less than 1	—	5	4	7	6	6	2	5	9	8
1 to 10	12	11	2	1	2	1	3	1	7	6
10 to 100	10	7	—	—	—	—	—	—	—	—
100 and over	1	—	—	—	—	—	—	—	—	—

*Number ($\times 10^6$) of asbestos fibers per gram of dried lung tissue in 76 male and 23 female patients with DMM in North America with matched controls. From reference 203.

Table 4-3

AMPHIBOLE FIBERS IN LUNG TISSUE OF 60 MALES WITH DIFFUSE MALIGNANT MESOTHELIOMA*

	Ever Employed	Either Amosite or Crocidolite	Amosite Only	Crocidolite Only
Heating trades	21	6	4	1
Shipyards	14	9	3	1
Construction	15	6	3	—
Insulation	8	6	1	—
Factory	2	2	2	—

*Amphibole fibers (more than a million per gram of dried lung tissue) in lung tissue of 60 men with mesothelioma ever employed in certain occupations. From reference 203.

and 3 controls had more than 1×10^6 fibers of anthophyllite and there were several cases with more than 10×10^6 fibers of tremolite. Although amosite is more common than crocidolite in the lungs of North Americans with DMM, both appear to be equally represented in the lungs of British DMM patients (203). When only one of these two asbestos types was present in the lung tissue of North American cases, it was almost always amosite (see Table 4-3).

It has been suggested that the carcinogenicity of chrysotile in relation to DMM may be due, at least in part, to contamination by tremolite asbestos (62); it was postulated that tremolite contamination may explain most cases of mesothelioma in the chrysotile mine workers of Quebec and perhaps in as many as 20 percent of the DMM cases occurring in the rest of Canada (205). However, a more recent report indicates that air contamination by tremolite may not be a significant determinant of DMM in Quebec chrysotile miners and millers (26). The incidence of mesothelioma in these workers was 62.5 per million per year from 1983 to 1990 (26). This is well above the rate for the general North American population, usually estimated at between 2.5 to 15 cases of DMM per year per million adult males (26). Very few cases of peritoneal DMM have been associated with chrysotile (89). Recent evidence associates anthophyllite with a few DMM cases in Finland (305).

The incidence of DMM rises with increasing intensity and duration of exposure to asbestos; the dose-specific risk data is in a linear relationship (89). There is no agreement on whether a threshold

of exposure exists, below which there is no risk of DMM. The incidence of DMM could be related to a power of time between three and four since exposure to asbestos first occurred (89).

There is marked variation in the reported extent of the association between asbestos exposure and DMM from one geographic area to another: a history of probable or definite exposure is seen in more than 70 percent of patients in some regions (331,347) and less than 30 percent in others (200,256). In 1972 in the United States, 64.8 percent of males with DMM had worked in occupations in which an association with asbestos was recognized (202). Asbestos exposure in some cases of mesothelioma has been slight (266) or of only a few months' duration (41,261); sometimes it has occurred in a nonoccupational setting (3). A further reflection of the low level of exposure in many patients, especially those with pleural DMM, is the absence of radiologic evidence of asbestos exposure (98) and the paucity of asbestos bodies and fibers in the lung parenchyma in some cases (251). Overall, our experience (205), and that reported in the recent literature, suggests that asbestos is causative in 70 to 90 percent of cases of DMM.

In assessing the results of studies on fiber burden in the lungs of DMM patients, it should be remembered that about 95 percent of the asbestos used in the past has been chrysotile, and that the fibers of this form of asbestos are broken up and cleared from the lung faster than those of other types of asbestos. Lung fiber counts may therefore substantially underestimate the extent of exposure to chrysotile, especially if the exposure

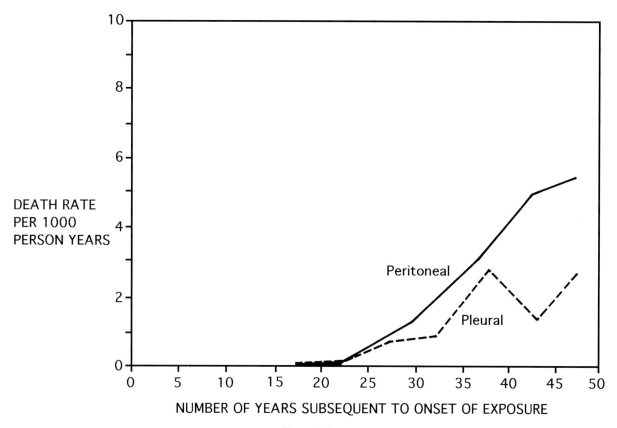

Figure 4-2

MESOTHELIOMA AND ASBESTOS EXPOSURE

Deaths per thousand person-years of experience by pleural and peritoneal mesotheliomas among 17,800 asbestos insulation workers from 1967 to 1976, analyzed by duration from onset of employment in 5-year periods. As of 45 years from onset, a decline in the mesothelioma rate is not noted. (Fig. 2 from Selikoff IJ, Hammond EC, Seidman H. Latency of asbestos disease among insulation workers in the United States and Canada. Cancer 1980;46:2737–40.)

occurred in the remote past. The amount of tremolite in lung tissue is probably a better marker of the extent of previous chrysotile inhalation (62). Lung tissue asbestos-body counts in DMM patients tend to be intermediate between those in the general population and those of patients with asbestosis (251). However, chrysotile asbestos does not form asbestos bodies as readily as does the amphiboles form of asbestos; asbestos bodies with a chrysotile fiber core account for only 2 percent of all asbestos bodies (251).

A latent period of 20 to 50 years, or even more, between the time of initial exposure to asbestos and the development of DMM is observed in most patients (average, 35 years) (fig. 4-2) (264). However, there have been rare instances when the latency interval has been much less than 20 years (28,58,83,125,234). Occasionally, DMM may occur in children (69,107,128,158,323).

It is generally believed that the pathogenesis of DMM involves migration of asbestos fibers to the affected serous membrane and physical contact between the fibers and mesothelial cells. The finding of fibers in the pleura (105) and in the substance of some peritoneal DMM cases (143) is consistent with this view. Chrysotile asbestos fibers migrate rapidly into the pleural cavity after intratracheal injection (307). Also, asbestos fibers rapidly penetrate the wall of the intestine (184), so that swallowing fibers cleared from the lung or directly ingesting fibers may contribute to their accumulation in the peritoneum. Lymphatic or hematogenous dissemination and passage through diaphragmatic stomata are other possible routes by which asbestos fibers might reach the peritoneum as well as other serous membranes and body tissues generally. Of interest is the experimental finding that pleural mesothelial cells may be stimulated by cytokines from asbestos-activated interstitial pulmonary macrophages that diffuse across the interstitium, without requiring translocation of fibers to the pleura (1).

Occasional mesothelial tumors appear to be induced by therapeutic radiation (118,186,285) or chronic inflammation (246). A synergistic effect between asbestos and some as yet unidentified environmental factors is also possible (251). Epidemiologic studies have shown no evidence of a relationship with smoking (201). DMM has been produced experimentally by various agents, including avian leukosis virus (54), diethylstilbestrol (189), and sterigmatocystin, a metabolite of molds that forms needle-like crystals (299). Recently, simian virus (SV40) has been shown to induce DMM when inserted into serosal cavities of hamsters (64). These findings, as well as the apparent absence of a history of significant asbestos exposure in 10 to 30 percent of human cases, implies that nonfibrous carcinogens and non-asbestiform fibers, including man-made mineral fibers, may have a role in causing mesothelioma in man as well as in animals. Although pleural fibrous plaques and other forms of pleural scarring are often seen radiologically or at autopsy in cases of pleural DMM, there is no convincing evidence that pleural scarring, per se, is involved in the pathogenesis of the tumor.

The association of asbestos exposure with carcinoma of the lung was demonstrated many years before the link between asbestos and DMM was recognized (207). It is clear that exposure to any of the commercial types of asbestos (chrysotile, amosite, crocidolite, tremolite, anthophyllite) may increase the risk of lung cancer. Cigarette smoke and asbestos synergize each other's carcinogenic effects in the lung; the potentiation appears to be multiplicative rather than additive (263). Although it has been suggested that asbestos exposure in nonsmokers does not increase the risk of lung carcinoma, evidence has emerged that asbestos has a measurable independent carcinogenic effect and that the relative risk in smoking and nonsmoking asbestos workers is similar (99,263). It has also been suggested that it is necessary for asbestos to produce interstitial pulmonary fibrosis (asbestosis) before an increased risk of lung cancer appears (40); in other studies, however, there seems to be an increased

Table 4-4

PATHOLOGIC EFFECTS OF ASBESTOS EXPOSURE IN MAN

Definite
Skin
  Asbestos corns
Lungs
  Diffuse interstitial fibrosis (asbestosis)
  Carcinoma following asbestosis
Pleura
  Diffuse mesothelioma
  Effusion
  Diffuse fibrosis in visceral pleura
  Fibrous plaques in parietal pleura
Peritoneum
  Diffuse mesothelioma

Probable
Larynx
  Carcinoma*
Pericardium and tunica vaginalis testis
  Diffuse mesothelioma (52,151)
Ovary
  Carcinoma (73,334)*
Gastrointestinal tract
  Carcinoma*

Possible
Lung
  Carcinoma without asbestosis (311)*
Reticuloendothelial system
  Lymphoma (114,150,255)*
Breast
  Carcinoma (92)*
Kidney
  Carcinoma (265)*
Pancreas
  Carcinoma (267)*
Peritoneum
  Serous surface papillary carcinoma of
    peritoneum (106)
  Well-differentiated papillary carcinoma of
    peritoneum (80,106)

---

* In these cases, the existence and strength of the association with asbestos has often been disputed in the literature and in the courts.

rate of lung cancer in the absence of asbestosis (311). The spectrum of carcinogenic and other effects of asbestos is summarized in Table 4-4.

Epidemiology. Although DMM remains an uncommon tumor, there is evidence of an increase in its frequency in some areas since 1950 (155,200). Because the frequency rate mainly reflects exposure to asbestos at least several decades previously and the use of asbestos continues to rise in some countries, upward trends in the overall incidence will probably continue. A further factor in this trend is the rapid increase in the risk of mesothelioma with the passage of time following the initial exposure (239). The incidence of DMM not related to commercial exposure to asbestos is 1 to 2 per million population per year (204). Projected estimates of the number of cases in the United States for the period 1980 to 2008 range from 19,000 to 79,000 (201). Males outnumber females several-fold in most studies, and according to some observers the increasing incidence is confined to males (201). DMM of pleural origin constitutes 65 to 75 percent of all malignant DMMs (201), although in several studies, workers heavily exposed to asbestos had a preponderance of peritoneal tumors (134,224). The incidence rates increase in each decade of life for both sexes (134), with occasional cases observed in childhood (69).

Insulation workers and those employed in certain asbestos processing plants and mines appear to be at particular risk. Table 4-5 lists occupational and other population groups associated with asbestos exposure. The relative risk for selected occupations is: insulators, 46.0; asbestos production and manufacture, 6.1; heating trades, 4.4; shipyard workers other than insulators, 2.8; construction industry, 2.6 (201). Those who reside with asbestos workers (domestic or household exposure) are also at increased risk (3,308), and secondary exposure in children may lead to the onset of DMM at an unusually early age. Transplacental transfer of asbestos may precipitate some cases of childhood DMM (323). Further forms of exposure arise from working in the same area as persons who are using asbestos (bystander or paraoccupational exposure) and from contamination of the environment (environmental or neighborhood exposure). Endemic pleural calcification and a high incidence of malignant mesothelioma from household use of asbestos have been reported in Metsovo, in northwestern Greece ("Metsovo lung"). In this and other areas of Greece, the occurrence of malignant mesothelioma has been attributed to use of a tremolite-containing whitewash (68).

Only a small percentage of women with DMM have been occupationally exposed (308). Familial occurrence has been reported, involving largely sibling-sibling or parent-child combinations (131, 247); occurrence in spousal pairs is rare (79).

Historically, asbestos-related disease was recognized as early as the 1920s and was associated with work in the mining and milling of asbestos ore and the manufacture of asbestos products (170). Initially, the number of patients was limited, but this was followed by a second phase which involved increasing numbers of workers using asbestos products, with a greater disease incidence. A third wave, due to "asbestos in place," has been widely recognized in recent years and stems from the aging and deterioration of buildings constructed with asbestos. This has created a serious potential for asbestos-related disease among persons engaged in the repair, renovation, and demolition of these buildings (170).

A history of exposure to asbestos or finding excess asbestos in the lungs is not evidence supporting the diagnosis of pleural DMM. It has been suggested that asbestos may cause as much as 5 percent of lung cancers (91) and may initiate several other forms of cancer (Table 4-4) (90).

Incidence in Various Serous Cavities. The relative frequency of peritoneal compared to pleural DMM has ranged from 1 to 10 to a preponderance in the peritoneum (98,134). Peritoneal mesothelioma is particularly common in insulation and asbestos factory workers (108, 134,224). Overall, peritoneal mesothelioma accounts for about a quarter of all cases of malignant mesothelioma (Table 4-6) (232). Approximately 2 percent of mesotheliomas arise in the pericardium, and a smaller number in the tunica vaginalis testis (206).

Clinical Features. Most malignant mesotheliomas develop in persons between the ages of 50 and 70 years (median, 50 to 60 years) (177). A few cases have been observed in the third and fourth decades, and, occasionally, children have been affected (128,323). Approximately 75 percent of reported cases occur in males (177). In North America and some other parts of the world, there has been a steady increase in the incidence of DMM in males in recent decades, whereas the incidence for females is unchanged (201).

The onset of pleural DMM is usually insidious. Chest pain and dyspnea are the most frequent initial complaints; cough, weight loss, and asthenia tend to develop somewhat later (98). Infrequently, DMM may present as recurrent pneumothorax (274), miliary dissemination in the absence of clinically identifiable pleural-based tumor (217), or enlargement of ipsilateral supraclavicular lymph nodes (289). The most distressing symptom as the disease progresses is pain

Table 4-5

USES OF AND EXPOSURES TO ASBESTOS*

Process/Product	Usage/Exposure	Groups Exposed
Asbestos mineral	Mining, milling, loading, or unloading	Miners, millers, dockers, truckers, etc. (O);*** individuals living near mines or mills (P,E)
Asbestos cement products	Cement pipes, sheets, other construction materials	Workers in manufacture (O); all workers engaged in building construction/demolition, including masons, plumbers, electricians, carpenters, welders (O)
Asbestos textiles	Fireproof cloth, lagging, curtains, padding	Workers in manufacture (O)
Asbestos floor tiles	Floor tile	Workers in manufacture/installation (O); general population (from normal wear) (E)
Asbestos friction products	Automotive brake/clutch linings	Workers in manufacture (O); automotive brake mechanics (O)
Asbestos paper products	Roofing and flooring felts, wallboard, insulating paper	Workers in manufacture (O); workers in installation (O); possible household contact (P,E)
Asbestos insulation products	Boiler/pipe installation; sprayed asbestos insulation (during construction or shipfitting/refitting; demolition/removal of asbestos insulation	Workers in manufacture (O); laggers, pipefitters, insulators, boilermakers (O); any type of construction/shipyard/railroad (steam)/demolition worker (O); welders, sheet metal workers, electricians, plumbers, and others who work near spraying or lagging (O); general population (from air contamination during removal or application (E)
	As insulation in public buildings	General population from slow liberation of fibers into air (E)
Miscellaneous products	Paints, plastics, filters, acoustic tiles, spackling, and similar products	Workers in manufacture/use (O); in beverages, IV drugs (E); in home repair (P)
Household contact exposure	Cleaning/washing contaminated work clothes	Close relatives of asbestos workers (P)
Environmental/building exposure	From commercial product liberated into air during construction/demolition; from commercial product liberated into buildings from ceilings/floors; from natural soil/rock-derived atmospheric/water contamination; from water contamination by dumping or use of asbestos cement pipe; from accidental use of asbestos-containing rock (for example, road paving) or accidental stirring up of asbestos rock/soil	General population (E)

*Modified from Table 7.5 in reference 60a.
**O = primarily occupational exposure; E = primarily environmental exposure; P = primarily paraoccupational exposure.

Table 4-6

DISTRIBUTION OF MALIGNANT MESOTHELIOMA BY SEX AND SITE, CANADA AND UNITED STATES*

	CANADA, 1960 to 1972			UNITED STATES, 1972		
	Males	**Females**	**Total**	**Males**	**Females**	**Total**
Pleural	155	62	217 (69.6%)	149	32	181 (73%)
Peritoneal	42	36	78 (25%)	32	19	51 (21%)
Pleural/Peritoneal	8	4	12 (3.9%)	6	3	9 (4%)
Pericardial	1	4	5 (1.5%)	2	2	4 (2%)
All sites	206 (66%)	106 (34%)	312 (100%)	189 (77%)	56 (23%)	245 (100%)

*In both the Canadian and US series, diagnosis was confirmed by autopsy in 64 percent and biopsy in 36 percent of cases. Table 6 from reference 206.

due to infiltration of the chest wall. The pain is often of an aching, nonpleuritic type and may be referred to the abdomen or shoulder. Evidence of pleural effusion is the most frequent finding on initial physical and radiographic examination (177,298), and a small proportion of DMMs are preceded for periods ranging from 1 to 7 years by recurrent pleural effusions. Close to 10 percent of patients have radiologic evidence of tumor without effusion (34). Asbestos workers may have recurrent pleural effusions with associated fibrous pleurisy (asbestos pleurisy) in the absence of any tumor (112). Chest roentgenogram and computerized tomographic (CT) scan may show a diffusely nodular or irregularly thickened pleura (figs. 4-3, 4-4), hilar or mediastinal masses, or masses of apparent pulmonary origin (136,278). The radiologic appearance may change markedly within a short time (fig. 4-5). Radiologic evidence of asbestosis is uncommon, whereas pleural plaques are seen quite frequently (98). Effusions are often blood stained, and may be massive and require frequent tapping. They tend to disappear in the later stages of the disease with advancing neoplastic thickening of the pleura and obliteration of the pleural cavity. Contraction of the affected hemithorax often occurs in the late stages, with pulling of the mediastinal structures to the affected side. Subcutaneous tumor nodules may appear in the chest wall, especially in relation to aspiration needle or thoracoscopy tracts and thoracotomy scars (98). The tumor may occasionally present as a mass in the chest wall or mimic Pancoast's tumor.

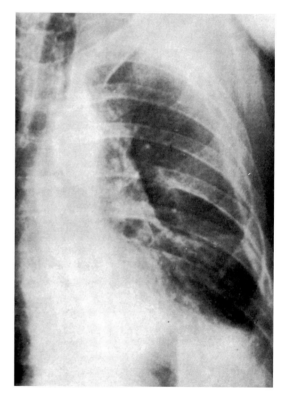

Figure 4-3

MALIGNANT MESOTHELIOMA

In this decubitus chest X ray, thick pleural "peel" surrounds the lung from apex to base. (Fig. 2-63 from Preger L. In: Asbestos-related disease. New York: Grune and Stratton, 1978:121–73.)

Extension of the neoplasm into the peritoneal and pericardial cavities, to the opposite pleural space, or to the mediastinum is fairly common in the later stages. The peritoneal cavity and one or both pleural cavities, may be involved at an early clinical stage. Although metastases are often found at

Figure 4-4
MALIGNANT
MESOTHELIOMA
In this CT scan, the pleura on the right side shows marked diffuse thickening by tumor. (Fig. 20 from Fascicle 20, 2nd Series.)

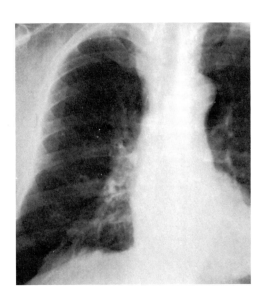
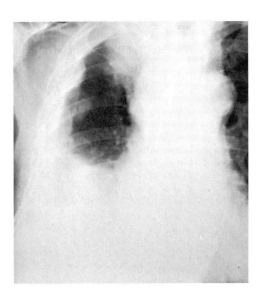

Figure 4-5
MALIGNANT MESOTHELIOMA
Rapid development of mesothelioma. The chest radiograph on the left is normal. Four months later, a large pleural-based mass encased the right lung. (Fig. 2-62 from Preger L. In: Asbestos-related disease. New York: Grune and Stratton, 1978:121–73.)

autopsy, they are seldom obvious during life. Digital clubbing and hypertrophic osteoarthropathy are uncommon. Hypoglycemia (144) and inappropriate secretion of antidiuretic and gonadotropic hormones (237,245) occur occasionally. The production of large amounts of interleu-

kin-6 by malignant mesothelioma has also been reported (139).

The clinical course of DMM of the peritoneum is even less specific than pleural DMM in its early stages. Abdominal discomfort or pain and gastrointestinal disturbances are common early

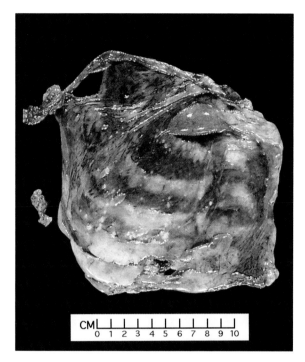

Figure 4-6
EARLY PLEURAL MESOTHELIOMA
Small isolated plaques of early invasive epithelial mesothelioma are visible. Much of the intervening pleural surface showed changes of mesothelioma in situ. (Courtesy of Dr. Douglas W. Henderson, Adelaide, Australia.)

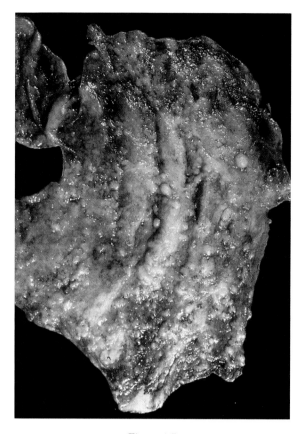

Figure 4-7
DIFFUSE PLEURAL MESOTHELIOMA
Confluent nodules of tumor on parietal pleura.

complaints. Ascites often occurs, and localized abdominal masses are sometimes palpable (153, 212). Intestinal obstruction frequently develops in the later stages. Evidence of extraperitoneal extension is unusual, but the tumor may first present in a hernia sac (225) or in remote lymph nodes (289). Thrombocytosis and thromboembolic episodes are common in large series of DMM (56). Imaging studies may show diffuse thickening of the peritoneum and mesentery, multiple small nodules, or a mass (252).

The average survival period of patients with diffuse pleural DMM from onset of symptoms is 12 to 15 months, and from the time of diagnosis, 8 to 12 months (178). However, considerably longer survival periods have been noted (331). The course of diffuse peritoneal DMM is often shorter than pleural DMM (98,153,212), but the rare cystic and well-differentiated papillary forms of the peritoneal tumor are less aggressive than pleural DMM (see pp. 49, 90). The therapeutic advances of recent years, especially in

chemotherapy, though limited, have increased the average survival period of DMM by several months. A few patients with diffuse pleural and peritoneal mesotheliomas have survived for 5 years or more (104,153,158,331,336).

Radiologic evidence of asbestos exposure is found in 50 percent of peritoneal DMM patients, but only in 12 percent with pleural DMM (98).

Gross Pathologic Findings. *Pleura.* In its early stages, as seen at thoracoscopy or thoracotomy, pleural DMM usually presents as multiple foci of tumor, often most prominent on the parietal pleura (36). These foci may take the form of innumerable tiny seedling-like deposits (fig. 4-6), or of a smaller number of more bulky, rounded, or plaque-like accumulations. With progression, the neoplastic foci become confluent (fig. 4-7), with resulting encasement of the lung and its individual lobes, and the residual pleural cavity, in a layer of tumor (fig. 4-8). The tumor is often

27

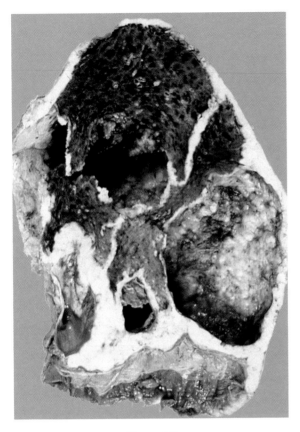

Figure 4-8
DIFFUSE PLEURAL MESOTHELIOMA

The lobes of the lung are encased by tumor. Parts of the pleural cavity persist as cystic locules. Note the thicker tumor rind at the base. (Fig. 13 from Hourihane DO, Mc-Caughey WT. Pathological aspects of asbestosis. Postgrad Med J 1966;42:612–3.)

nodular where it borders residual effusion fluid (fig. 4-7). The tumor may reach several centimeters in thickness, especially basally, and, on occasion, prominent masses form in a diffuse tumor. As the bulk of the neoplasm increases, the pleural cavity becomes progressively obliterated, but even in advanced cases, parts of the cavity may persist as cystic locules filled with viscous fluid or jelly-like material. Localized malignant mesotheliomas, including epithelioid and biphasic histologic types, and sessile and pedunculated forms, may occasionally occur (74,342).

What appears to be an adhesive fibrous pleurisy of non-neoplastic nature at thoracotomy or autopsy may be found to be an early DMM on microscopic examination. Rarely, cystic spaces, usually small, may be seen grossly in the substance of pleural DMM.

Widespread extension into the soft tissues of the chest wall is often noted in the later stages of the disease, and the tumor may sometimes penetrate extensively into subcutaneous tissue, especially when needle or drainage tube tracts or scars are present. Mediastinal involvement, with invasion of the pericardial sac and sometimes the heart, and encirclement of other mediastinal structures, is also common (fig. 4-9) Infiltration of the diaphragm is a frequent finding, and some degree of peritoneal involvement is found in at least one third of autopsied cases. Often, the peritoneal dissemination is localized mainly to the upper abdomen on the side of the pleural tumor, but is sometimes so extensive that it is difficult, on the basis of the autopsy findings alone, to be sure of the cavity of origin. Spread to the opposite pleural cavity through the mediastinum is not uncommon. Rarely, contemporaneous involvement of two serous cavities is seen at an early disease stage, or even as its initial manifestation.

Superficial invasion of the ipsilateral lung is often noted at autopsy. In some cases, however, there is more extensive involvement of the pulmonary parenchyma in the form of a large mass, multiple nodules, or extensive replacement of a lobe. Rarely, an otherwise typical DMM surrounds or infiltrates the wall of a major bronchus at the pulmonary hilus. Dissemination through both lungs in the manner of a lymphangitis carcinomatosa is seen terminally in many papillary or tubulopapillary epithelial DMMs (fig. 4-10).

Occasionally, poorly circumscribed, bulky pleural tumors impinge on a large area of serosa because of their size rather than by permeation or seeding. Also, a malignant serosal neoplasm may be found at such an early stage that its potential for diffuse involvement of the pleura is not obvious. Such tumors may be categorized justifiably as malignant mesothelioma on microscopic grounds, but it is better for therapeutic and epidemiologic reasons to reserve the designation "diffuse" for tumors that show a clear-cut predilection to spread or scatter in or along the serous membranes.

Pleural DMM frequently metastasizes to mediastinal lymph nodes and at times to abdominal, cervical, or axillary nodes. Although hematogenous dissemination to remote viscera was once thought to be rare, experience has shown that this form of metastasis is found at autopsy

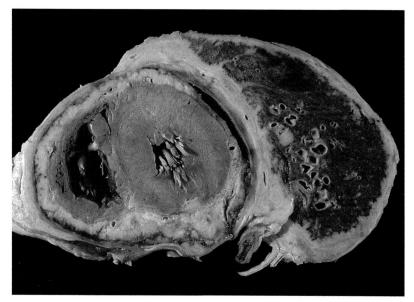

Figure 4-9
DIFFUSE PLEURAL
MESOTHELIOMA
Extensive involvement of the pericardium. (Courtesy of Dr. Samuel Hammar, Seattle, WA.)

Figure 4-10
DIFFUSE PLEURAL
MESOTHELIOMA
Extensive intrapulmonary lymphangitic spread.

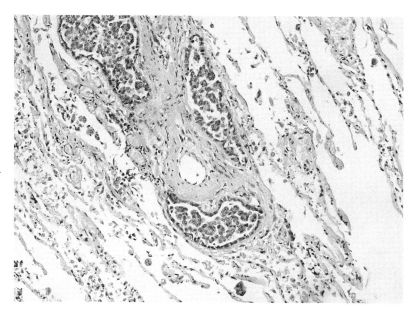

in one third to half of mesotheliomas (51,98,249). Blood-borne metastases occur more commonly with sarcomatous mesothelial tumors (fig. 4-11) and their desmoplastic variants than with nonsarcomatous types (51). Lung, liver, kidney, adrenal gland, and bone are the most common sites for blood-borne metastases, but other viscera, including intestine, brain, and thyroid, are occasionally involved.

Peritoneum. When the tumor originates in the abdominal cavity, the serosal surface often becomes studded with myriads of nodules of varying size, indistinguishable from those of carcinomatosis peritonei (fig. 4-12). Intestinal adhesions and nodularity or induration of the omentum may appear at an early stage. Massive accumulations of tumor, up to 25 cm in diameter, may sometimes occur, especially in the omentum, lower abdominal cavity, and pelvis (153). Plaques of confluent growth and diffuse peritoneal thickening are frequently seen. In the late stages, as found at autopsy, encasement of the liver and

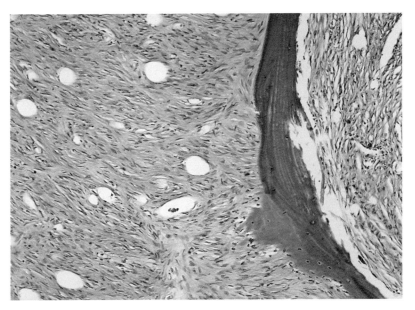

Figure 4-11
DIFFUSE MESOTHELIOMA,
DESMOPLASTIC TYPE
Metastasis to vertebral bone. Note the bland appearance of the tumor cells, simulating a low-grade fibrosarcoma.

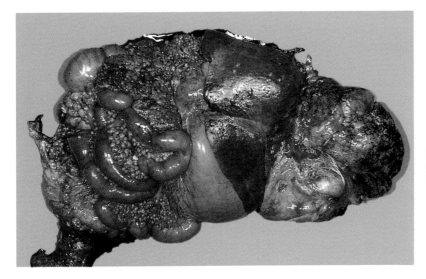

Figure 4-12
DIFFUSE PERITONEAL
MESOTHELIOMA
Confluent nodules and hepatic metastases are noted. The gross appearance is indistinguishable from peritoneal carcinomatosis.

spleen, and extensive visceral adhesions are often present. The viscera may eventually become completely encased in tumor and the peritoneal cavity obliterated (fig. 4-13).

Invasion of underlying tissues is noted in about one third of peritoneal DMMs. Usually, this is seen in the omentum and the outer parts of the wall of the gastrointestinal tract. Infiltration of the liver capsule is also common. Less frequently, retroperitoneal tissues are invaded by tumor, and the kidney or pancreas may be surrounded. Occasionally, extension into the pancreas is noted. Although the undersurface of the diaphragm is often studded with tumor, the diaphragmatic muscle is seldom invaded. It is rare for a mesothelioma originating in the peritoneum to spread to the pleural cavity, although the reverse situation is common in advanced pleural DMM. Occasionally, combined pleural and peritoneal involvement may be seen at a relatively early stage of the disease. In this situation, it may be impossible to determine on a pathologic basis which cavity was primarily involved. Although extension to the tunica vaginalis testis occurs infrequently (153), it may be the initial manifestation (225). Invasion of the abdominal wall is uncommon and is usually related to a laparotomy or laparoscopy scar.

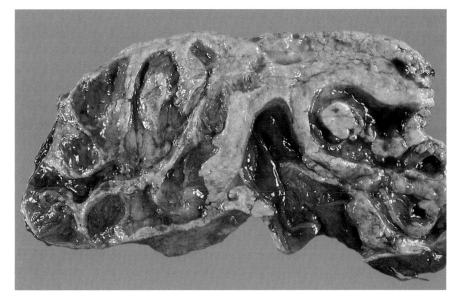

Figure 4-13
DIFFUSE PERITONEAL
MESOTHELIOMA
Loops of intestine are completely encased by tumor.

Metastases are observed in 50 percent of autopsy cases (153). They usually involve abdominal lymph nodes, but may also occur in inguinal, thoracic, and axillary lymph nodes; liver; lung; and, uncommonly, other sites.

Tunica Vaginalis Testis. Malignant mesothelioma of the tunica vaginalis consists of multiple nodules or papillary excrescences which stud the serosal surface of the tunica and which may eventually encase the scrotal contents. Cystic spaces may be seen in the tumor (313). The tumor may extend to the peritoneal surfaces and involve retroperitoneal lymph nodes (5).

Pericardium. The gross characteristics of DMM in this site are described in Fascicle 15, Second Series, Tumors of the Cardiovascular System (190). The tumors progress to encase the heart and the attachments of major vessels. The myocardium is often focally invaded, but unlike many primary cardiac sarcomas, the tumor does not involve the endocardium or enter a heart chamber. Spread to adjacent pleura and the mediastinum is frequently noted and, in a few cases, there may be extension into the peritoneal cavity and involvement of mediastinal lymph nodes. Pleural DMM frequently spreads to the pericardial sac (fig. 4-9).

Microscopic Findings. In spite of the relatively stereotypic gross characteristics and behavior, DMMs have a diversity of cytoarchitectural characteristics that are almost unique among neoplasms originating from a single cell line. The spectrum embraces tumors that are entirely of epithelial or mesenchymal type to a range of biphasic and intermediate forms. Moreover, as with other malignant neoplasms, cellular and architectural forms may vary from well-differentiated to anaplastic. Several cytoarchitectural patterns associated with the tumor are highly specific; others are common to many types of cancer, and histochemical, immunohistochemical, and ultrastructural studies are often required to confirm the diagnosis.

Four main histologic categories of DMM are recognized: epithelial (tubulopapillary and epithelioid), sarcomatous (including desmoplastic), biphasic (mixed), and poorly differentiated (or undifferentiated). Fifty percent of pleural DMMs and 75 percent of peritoneal DMMs are of epithelial type (153); 25 and 15 percent, respectively, are of biphasic and sarcomatous types; and the remaining cases are poorly differentiated or unclassifiable. The proportion of tumors in the latter category being classified into a "probable" or "definite" DMM group depends on the nature and extent of exclusionary investigations (clinical or at autopsy) and the availability of immunohistochemical and ultrastructural studies (76). The existence of the poorly differentiated group has been ignored in many reports, which may, in turn, have led to a significant underestimation of the frequency of DMM.

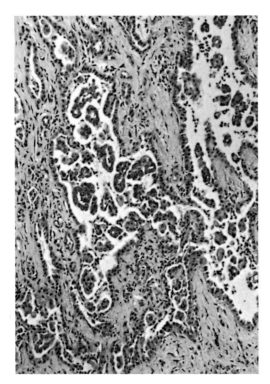

Figure 4-14
DIFFUSE MESOTHELIOMA, EPITHELIAL TYPE
Papillae, branching spaces, and tubules are lined by cuboidal epithelium in this mesothelioma of tubulopapillary pattern (X125). (Fig. 34 from Fascicle 20, 2nd Series.)

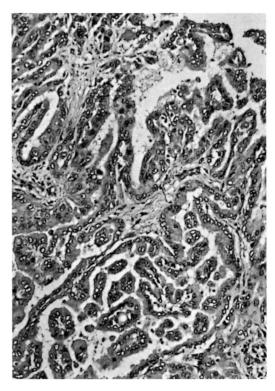

Figure 4-15
DIFFUSE MESOTHELIOMA, EPITHELIAL TYPE
This tubulopapillary pattern shows tumor cell nuclei that are quite regular and markedly vesicular (X200). (Fig. 35 from Fascicle 20, 2nd Series.)

Diagnosis of biphasic tumors depends on the amount of tissue available and the extent to which it is sampled. Precise diagnostic criteria, particularly the minimum amounts of the two phenotypic components required, have not been defined. There is sometimes a high degree of subjectivity involved in determining whether the proliferating spindle cell component of a putative biphasic mesothelioma represents cellular stroma or sarcoma (sarcoma-like). Application of the word "epithelioid" is also subject to observer variation. Such factors may account for some of the differences in the frequency of biphasic and sarcomatous mesotheliomas reported in the literature. Sarcomatous mesothelioma rarely occurs in the peritoneum in our own experience and that of others (153).

The histologic characteristics of DMM have been detailed in a number of reports and texts (17,157,192,196). Epithelial DMM is usually tubulopapillary (figs. 4-14, 4-15), but predominantly tubular or papillary patterns are sometimes seen (figs. 4-16, 4-17). The tumor cells in well-differentiated tubulopapillary neoplasms often have acidophilic cytoplasm, are usually cuboidal or flattened, and sometimes possess relatively uniform vesicular nuclei with prominent nucleoli. A microcystic pattern is present in a small proportion of cases (fig. 4-18) and rarely, larger cystic areas are present (fig. 4-19). Macrocystic mesothelial tumors (benign cystic mesothelioma or multilocular inclusion cysts) sometimes arise from the peritoneum (see p. 90), or, occasionally, from the pleura (13). Rarely, there are areas that resemble an angiosarcoma (fig. 4-20) or an epithelioid hemangioendothelioma.

In areas of the tubular or tubulopapillary form, tumor cells are low columnar or columnar and show marked pleomorphism in size, shape, and nuclear characteristics; they resemble adenocarcinoma in various stages of differentiation (figs. 4-21, 4-22). A form of primary serous papillary carcinoma of

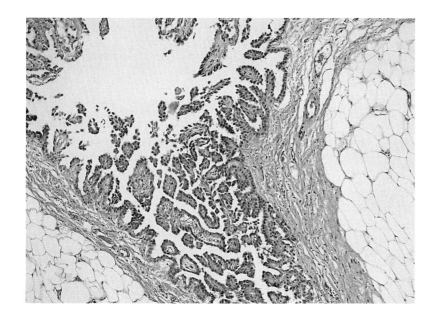

Figure 4-16
DIFFUSE MESOTHELIOMA,
EPITHELIAL TYPE
Predominantly papillary.

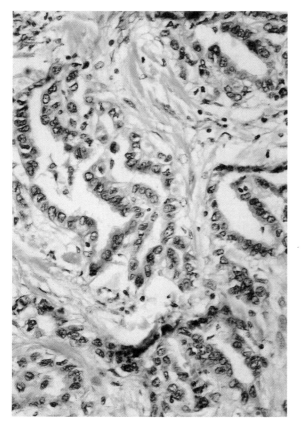

Figure 4-17
DIFFUSE MESOTHELIOMA, EPITHELIAL TYPE
Predominant tubular pattern.

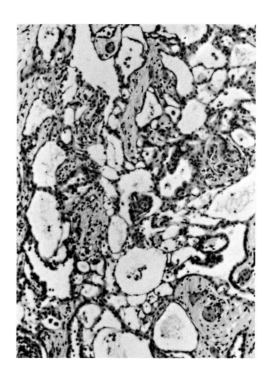

Figure 4-18
DIFFUSE MESOTHELIOMA, MICROCYSTIC PATTERN
Numerous small cystic spaces are lined by cuboidal or flat-
tened tumor cells (X125). (Fig. 39 from Fascicle 20, 2nd Series.)

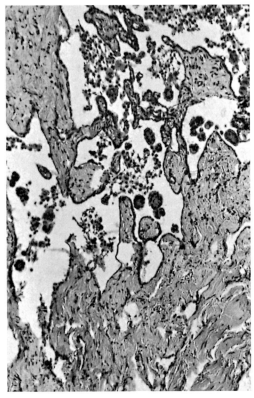

Figure 4-19
DIFFUSE MESOTHELIOMA, CYSTIC TYPE

The large space contains papillary ingrowths. Parts of the tumor were noted to be cystic, grossly. The appearance is similar to that of a vascular neoplasm (X50). (Fig. 38 from Fascicle 20, 2nd Series.)

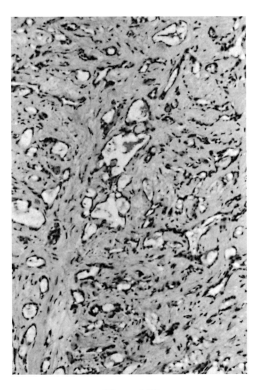

Figure 4-20
DIFFUSE MESOTHELIOMA, EPITHELIAL TYPE

Small branching tubules lined by markedly flattened cells are dispersed through a dense fibrous stroma. This degree of flattening of neoplastic mesothelium is unusual and gives the tumor an angiomatous appearance (X125). (Fig. 31 from Fascicle 20, 2nd Series.)

Figure 4-21
MESOTHELIOMA
RESEMBLING CARCINOMA

The appearance is similar to that of adenocarcinoma, but the prominent cytoplasmic vacuoles did not stain with mucicarmine (X125). (Fig. 42 from Fascicle 20, 2nd Series.)

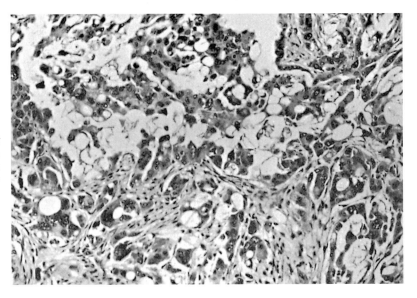

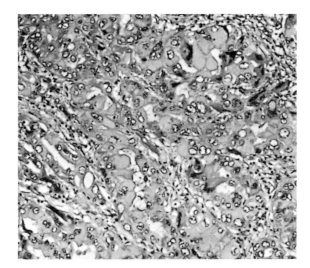

Figure 4-22
MESOTHELIOMA RESEMBLING CARCINOMA
A histologic distinction between adenocarcinoma and
mesothelioma is impossible in areas such as this. Diagnosis
must usually be based on the gross anatomic findings, the
presence or absence microscopically of areas more typical of
mesothelioma, and the results of staining for epithelial
mucin (X200). (Fig. 41 from Fascicle 20, 2nd Series.)

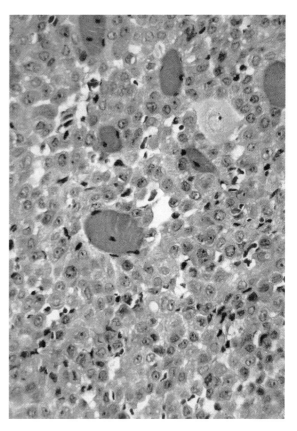

Figure 4-23
DIFFUSE MESOTHELIOMA, EPITHELIAL TYPE
In this predominantly solid type, bland-appearing tumor
cells were initially interpreted as hyperplastic mesothelium.
The tumor recurred at the biopsy site. Skeletal muscle cells
are surrounded by the invading tumor.

the peritoneum, histologically similar to primary
serous papillary carcinoma of the ovary, has been
noted in women; a well-differentiated papillary
DMM of the peritoneum that occurs mainly in
women, and often behaves in a benign fashion,
has also been observed (see p. 49).

There is a solid (nonglandular) form of epithelial DMM (*epithelioid mesothelioma*) which is
composed of clumps or sheets of plump round or
polyhedral cells with voluminous acidophilic cytoplasm, best seen in hematoxylin and eosin–
stained preparations. When well differentiated,
the cells may closely resemble hyperplastic mesothelium and pose a difficult diagnostic problem in small biopsies (fig. 4-23). In this solid or
epithelioid form, the cells may also show considerable nuclear pleomorphism, with giant cells
occasionally present (fig. 4-24). Large cytoplasmic vacuoles that do not stain with periodic
acid–Schiff (PAS) may be conspicuous (fig. 4-25);
and the vacuoles may become confluent and
stimulate a giant cell reaction (fig. 4-26). The
term *transitional mesothelioma* refers to a histologic type of DMM having features transitional or
intermediate between epithelial DMM and sarcomatoid mesothelioma (fig. 4-27) (132,196). It has

been suggested that some mesotheliomas designated as "poorly differentiated" by others (78) fit
in the transitional mesothelioma category (134).
If a poorly differentiated mesothelioma has substantial areas where the tumor cells are of intermediate (or transitional) character as defined
above, it is appropriate to include it in the transitional group, irrespective of the cell size and
nuclear characteristics. Squamous metaplasia,
although rare, may be seen in otherwise bona
fide mesothelioma (169). A small cell variant of
DMM has been described (187) (see p. 49).

The stroma in epithelial DMM tumors varies
in amount. It may be dense or loosely formed and
moderately cellular. On occasion, the stroma has
a distinctive edematous or myxoid appearance
(fig. 4-28) which is rarely, if ever, seen in adenocarcinomas. A diffuse lymphoid inflammatory

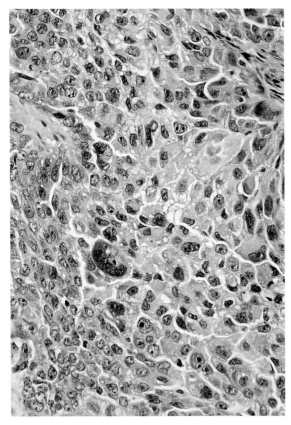

Figure 4-24
DIFFUSE MESOTHELIOMA, EPITHELIAL TYPE
Pleomorphism and formation of giant cells are evident.

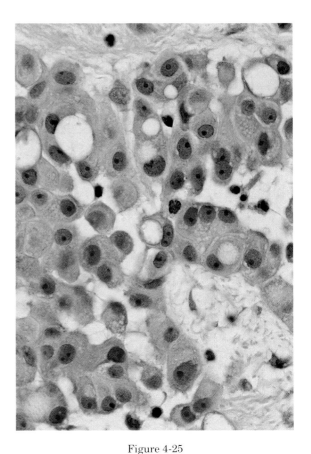

Figure 4-25
DIFFUSE MESOTHELIOMA, EPITHELIAL TYPE
Numerous intracytoplasmic vacuoles, some of which are large, are present. These failed to stain with the PAS and mucicarmine stains.

Figure 4-26
VACUOLATION IN MESOTHELIOMA
Large cytoplasmic vacuoles are becoming confluent. The vacuoles did not stain with PAS or with Meyer's mucicarmine stain. The material in the vacuoles has caused a giant cell reaction (X125). (Fig. 55 from Fascicle 20, 2nd Series.)

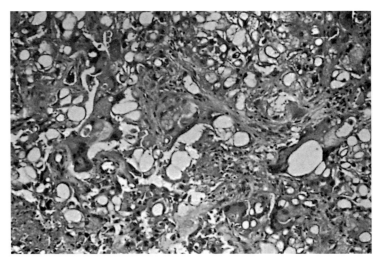

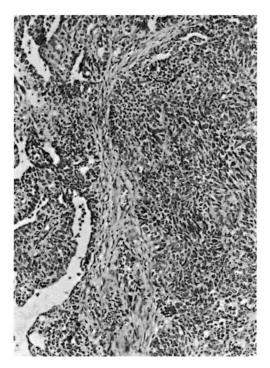

Figure 4-27
DIFFUSE MESOTHELIOMA, INTERMEDIATE CELLS
Irregular spaces lined by mesothelioma cells are seen at left. The sheet of cells on the right has an appearance intermediate between a sarcoma and a carcinoma (X125). (Fig. 76 from Fascicle 20, 2nd Series.)

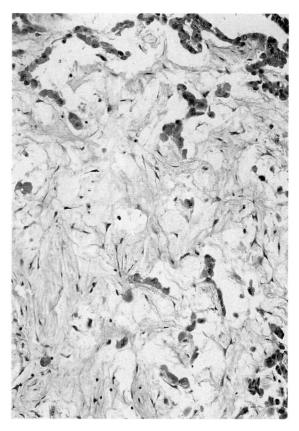

Figure 4-28
DIFFUSE MESOTHELIOMA, EPITHELIAL TYPE
Myxoid stroma.

cell infiltrate is noted in a small number of DMMs and is characteristic of the rare lymphohistiocytoid variant (see fig. 4-49). When the stroma is cellular, it is difficult to decide if it is stroma or a sarcomatous component of a biphasic tumor.

In tumors that are entirely or partly sarcomatous, the neoplastic mesenchymal tissue is composed of spindle-shaped or oval cells (fig. 4-29) and may have a variety of histologic patterns. Giant cells are occasionally prominent (fig. 4-30). For the most part, the patterns of the tumor cells are nonspecific and overlap with those of a number of soft tissue tumors including malignant fibrous histiocytoma, malignant schwannoma, fibrous sarcoma, and rhabdomyosarcoma. Storiform or interweaving patterns are not uncommon (fig. 4-31), but a well-developed fascicular pattern is rare. In occasional cases, foci identical to malignant osteoid or cartilage may be seen in sarcomatous mesothelioma or sarcomatous areas of biphasic mesothelioma (figs. 4-32, 4-33). (345). Rarely, small numbers of psammoma bodies are

found in tubulopapillary mesothelioma (fig. 4-34) (126). Heavy calcification of metastatic tumor in the liver has been described (50,238). A diffuse myxochondrosarcoma of the pleura has been reported (122).

In the desmoplastic form of diffuse mesothelioma, much of the tumor is fibrous and may be difficult to distinguish from reactive pleural fibrosis (fig. 4-35). Desmoplastic mesothelioma is usually associated with the presence of obvious sarcomatous elements in at least some part of the tumor; epithelial elements may also be present (51). Desmoplastic areas in a DMM may resemble banal scar tissue or assume a more distinctive whorled or storiform pattern; they may be paucicellular, but usually show at least some degree of nuclear atypia (fig. 4-36). When DMM of the sarcomatous or fibrous type invades the lung, the tumor cells at the advancing margin often fill the alveolar spaces in a distinctive way (figs. 4-37, 4-38). Infrequently, DMM will invade the alveolar septa (fig. 4-39).

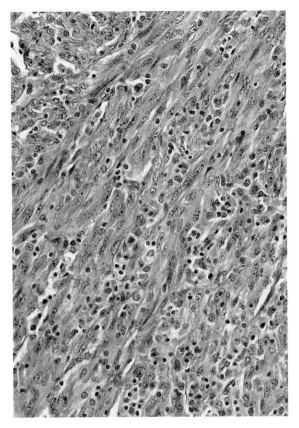

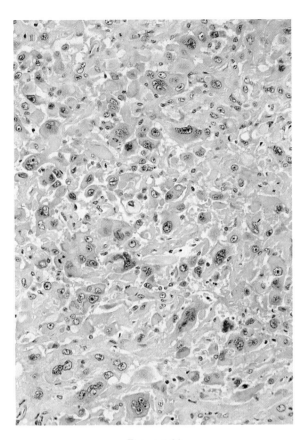

Figure 4-29
DIFFUSE SARCOMATOUS MESOTHELIOMA
Predominant spindle-shaped tumor cells mimicking leiomyosarcoma or fibrosarcoma.

Figure 4-30
DIFFUSE SARCOMATOUS MESOTHELIOMA
Numerous tumor giant cells confer an appearance reminiscent of malignant fibrous histiocytoma.

Figure 4-31
DIFFUSE SARCOMATOUS
MESOTHELIOMA
Prominent storiform pattern of growth in a pleural mesothelioma from an asbestos worker. (Periodic acid–Schiff stain)

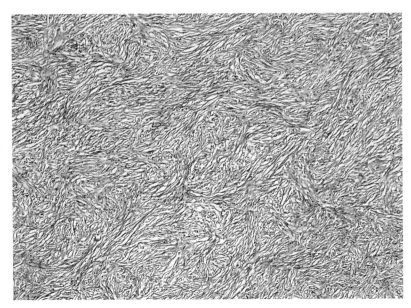

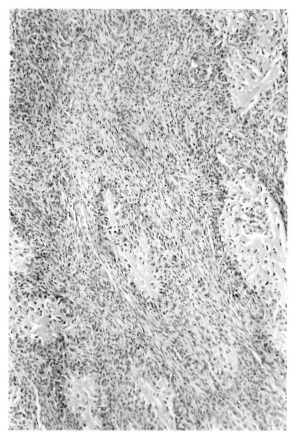

Figure 4-32
DIFFUSE SARCOMATOUS MESOTHELIOMA
Several foci of malignant osteoid tissue are present.

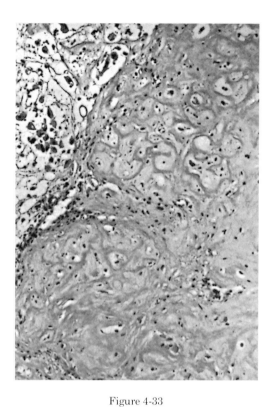

Figure 4-33
CARTILAGINOUS METAPLASIA
IN MESOTHELIOMA
The tumor has a cartilaginous character in this area
(X125). (Fig. 50 from Fascicle 20, 2nd Series.)

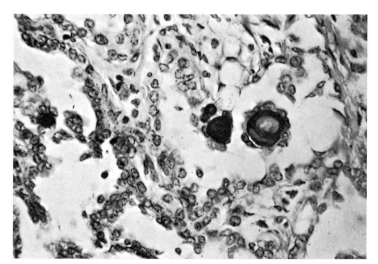

Figure 4-34
PSAMMOMA BODIES
IN MESOTHELIOMA
Psammoma bodies are present in this well-
differentiated epithelial mesothelioma. These
bodies are rarely found in mesotheliomas
(X350). (Fig. 51 from Fascicle 20, 2nd Series.)

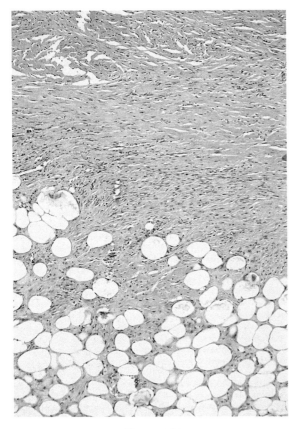

Figure 4-35
DIFFUSE SARCOMATOUS MESOTHELIOMA
This was initially misdiagnosed as fibrous pleuritis. Note invasion of the adipose tissue of the parietal pleura by bland fibroblast-like cells.

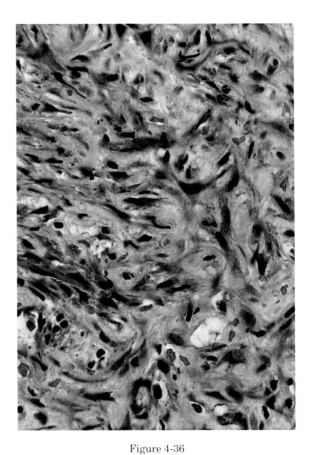

Figure 4-36
DIFFUSE SARCOMATOUS MESOTHELIOMA
Another field from same tumor as shown in figure 4-27 showing an area of moderate cell atypia. These areas were, however, infrequent in this tumor.

Figure 4-37
INVASION OF ALVEOLI
The tumor cells at the advancing margin of this sarcomatous mesothelioma fill the alveolar spaces. This pattern is frequently seen when sarcomatous mesotheliomas invade lung (X48). (Fig. 68 from Fascicle 20, 2nd Series.)

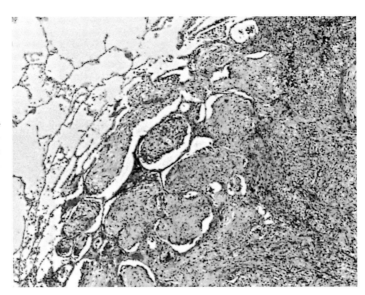

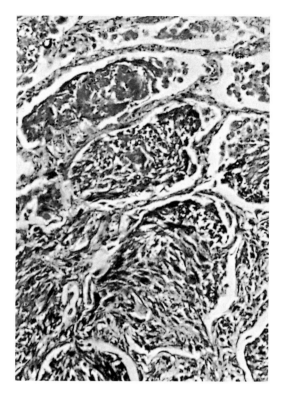

Figure 4-38
INVASION OF ALVEOLI
Tumor cells admixed with fibrin occupy the alveolar spaces. There is a superficial resemblance to an organizing pneumonia (X125). (Fig. 69 from Fascicle 20, 2nd Series.)

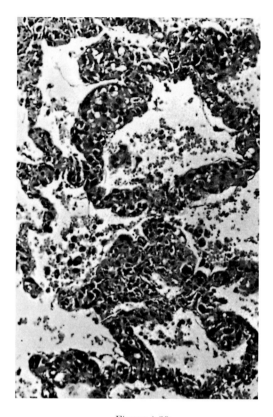

Figure 4-39
INVASION OF ALVEOLAR SEPTA
Tumor is infiltrating the alveolar septa diffusely (X125). (Fig. 71 from Fascicle 20, 2nd Series.)

In biphasic tumors, malignant elements of both epithelial and mesenchymal appearance are present. Frequently the two phenotypes occur in different parts of the same tumor, but sometimes they are intimately admixed (fig. 4-40). Cells of the intermediate or transitional type are commonly seen in association with tubulopapillary or tubular forms of the tumor (see fig. 4-27).

In its poorly differentiated or undifferentiated form, DMM is usually composed of sheets of plump or polygonal cells, which may show considerable nuclear pleomorphism (fig. 4-41). Careful search sometimes reveals cells whose appearance is similar to that of epithelioid DMM cells, but differentiation from carcinoma requires ultrastructural, immunohistochemical, and various exclusionary studies (76). Occasional undifferentiated pleural DMM shows prominent clear cell areas, making it very difficult to distinguish from clear cell carcinoma originating in the kidney or elsewhere (fig. 4-42) (195). Two very unusual cases have been reported in which metastatic cancer was mimicked by mesothelial cell inclusions in mediastinal lymph nodes. Both patients had pleuritis with pleural effusion (38).

Unusual Variants. A number of unusual histologic variants of DMM are recognized and are listed in Table 4-7.

Desmoplastic Mesothelioma. This variant of DMM has been arbitrarily categorized as a tumor in which more than 50 percent is poorly cellular, dense fibrous tissue (51,138,335). Desmoplastic mesothelioma constitutes 10 percent of all DMMs (335); most are pleural (51). Seventy percent of patients with desmoplastic mesothelioma have had previous occupational exposure to asbestos (335).

The appearance of the fibrous areas of desmoplastic mesothelioma vary considerably. Some may be nondescript, with laminar hyaline collagen

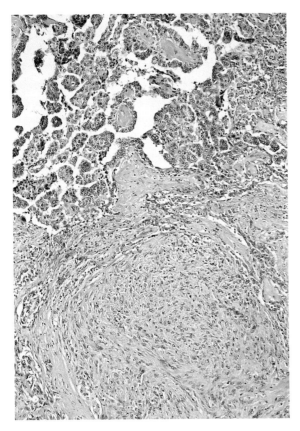 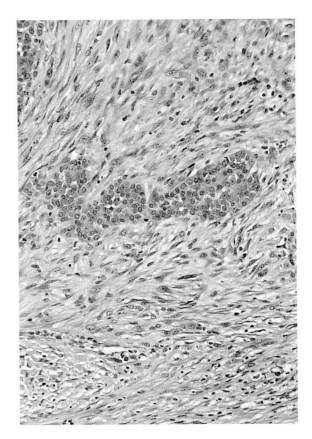

Figure 4-40
BIPHASIC MALIGNANT MESOTHELIOMA
Left: Site of coexistence of epithelial and sarcomatous phases.
Right: Small focus of epithelial mesothelioma in a predominantly sarcomatous mesothelioma.

Table 4-7

**UNUSUAL VARIANTS OF DIFFUSE
MALIGNANT MESOTHELIOMA**

Desmoplastic mesothelioma

Lymphohistiocytoid mesothelioma

Small cell mesothelioma

Mesothelioma in situ

Well-differentiated papillary mesothelioma

Malignant mesothelioma of tunica vaginalis

Localized mesothelioma

Deciduoid peritoneal mesothelioma

accompanied by small numbers of flattened cells (fig. 4-43). However, the neoplastic nature of these areas is indicated by the presence of more cellular foci in which there is considerable nuclear irregularity and hyperchromasia. Other fibrous parts of the tumor have a more distinctive pattern, with branching bands or wire-like strands of acidophilic hyaline collagen forming whorls, interweaving fascicles, complex meshworks, and storiform foci (fig. 4-44). These patterns are rarely seen in inflammatory scarring and should alert the observer to the likely existence of desmoplastic mesothelioma. The cellularity in such areas is variable. A basket-weave pattern, similar to that seen in pleural plaque, is sometimes present; this pattern blends with other fibrous elements, suggesting that it is an integral part of the neoplasm rather than the remains of a preexisting fibrous plaque that was

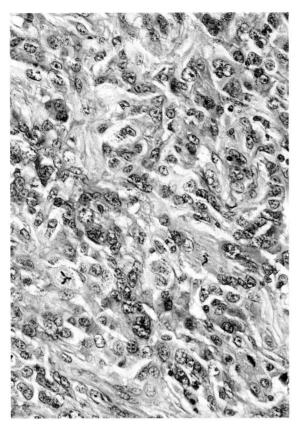

Figure 4-41
POORLY DIFFERENTIATED MESOTHELIOMA
Marked pleomorphism, atypical mitoses, and an indistinct pattern of growth are common in this type.

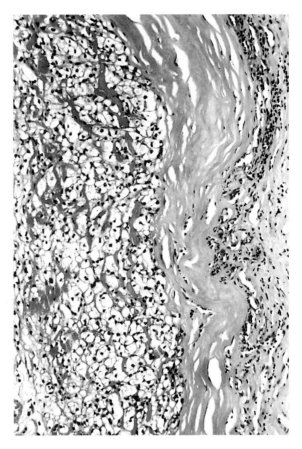

Figure 4-42
DIFFUSE MESOTHELIOMA, EPITHELIAL TYPE
Presence of abundant clear cells give the tumor a histologic appearance reminiscent of clear cell carcinoma of the kidney.

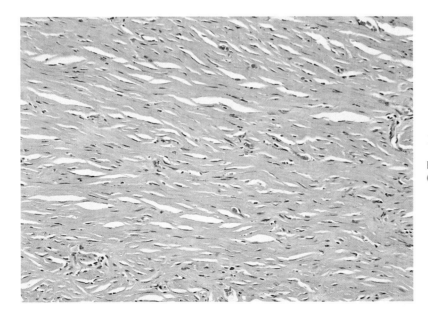

Figure 4-43
DESMOPLASTIC MESOTHELIOMA
This pleural-based tumor, despite its bland appearance, metastasized to bone (compare with figure 4-11).

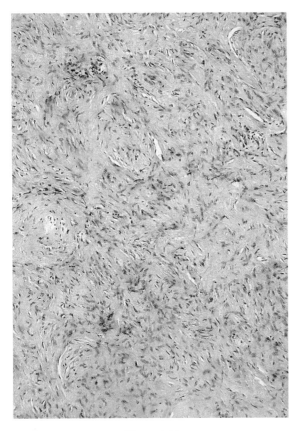

Figure 4-44
DESMOPLASTIC MESOTHELIOMA
Storiform pattern of growth.

incorporated in the tumor. At times, cellular granulation tissue with no specific characteristics forms a continuous zone adjacent to the residual pleural cavity (fig. 4-45). When, as is often the case, the fibrous areas of the tumor are mainly hypocellular, it is the nuclear atypia seen in more structured areas of the desmoplastic mesothelioma that suggests the process is neoplastic and not reactive.

Nodules of fibrous tumor sometimes infiltrate alveolar spaces in the adjacent lung or the soft tissues of the chest wall. In most instances, cellular areas with sarcomatous characteristics can be found in parts of the tumor, although a careful search is sometimes necessary. In about one third of cases, epithelial-type tumor elements, usually of tubular or papillary form, are seen at least focally (fig. 4-46) and may be accompanied by obvious sarcomatous areas. Zones of bland infarct-like necrosis are quite common. As such

zones are rarely seen in inflammatory fibrosis, they help to distinguish desmoplastic mesothelioma from fibrous pleurisy. It has been suggested that the most cellular tissue found in desmoplastic mesothelioma is at the mediastinal aspect of the pleura (138). A feature frequently seen in desmoplastic mesothelioma and rarely, if ever, in fibrosing pleuritis is focal invasion into the underlying pulmonary parenchyma along interlobular septa and fissures and into subserosal adipose tissue in the parietal pleura (fig. 4-47). Such areas of focal invasion may be made apparent by immunostaining with antibodies to low molecular weight cytokeratins (fig. 4-48)(17). Nonetheless, even when abundant decortication material is available, and numerous samples are taken, confident differentiation between desmoplastic mesothelioma and fibrous pleurisy may be difficult or impossible. It should be remembered that there are many causes of benign diffuse pleural fibrosis, one of which is asbestos (112). Asbestos is also the main cause of the discrete fibrous plaques that are frequently seen on the parietal pleura in persons exposed to asbestos.

In cases in which only small biopsy specimens are available, localized malignant fibrous tumors of the pleura (so-called malignant localized mesothelioma) may enter into the differential diagnosis because of the dense fibrosis that occurs in some of them. Immunostaining for low molecular weight keratins helps in diagnosis since desmoplastic mesotheliomas nearly always express keratin, whereas benign localized fibrous tumors do not. Ultrastructurally, desmoplastic mesothelioma is similar to conventional sarcomatoid mesothelioma, but with more cells with the appearance of myofibroblasts (75). However, the frequent expression of cytokeratins by the cells of desmoplastic mesothelioma sets them apart from myofibroblasts (17,100).

Lymphohistiocytoid Mesothelioma. This form of DMM is characterized by large histiocyte-like tumor cells and a diffuse, often fairly heavy, lymphocytic infiltration of the substance of the tumor (fig. 4-49)(137,138). Plasma cells and eosinophils may also be noted in the cellular infiltrate. This variant of DMM may be confused with malignant lymphoma (138). Grossly, the tumor forms multiple pleural nodules. The large histiocyte-like tumor cells are round or oval, and possess moderate amounts of pale acidophilic cytoplasm, nuclei

Figure 4-45
DESMOPLASTIC MESOTHELIOMA
Left: In this section near the pleural surface, the tumor blends imperceptibly with granulation tissue (upper field).
Right: Parallel section stained with a cocktail of monoclonal antibodies to low molecular weight keratins. Note the intense reactivity of the tumor cells and absence of staining of the granulation tissue.

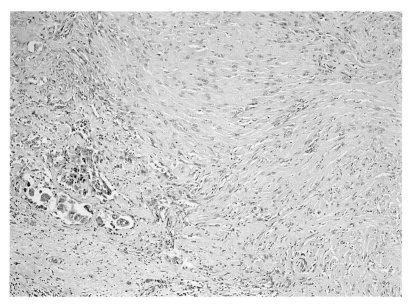

Figure 4-46
DESMOPLASTIC MESOTHELIOMA
Small focus of epithelial mesothelioma.

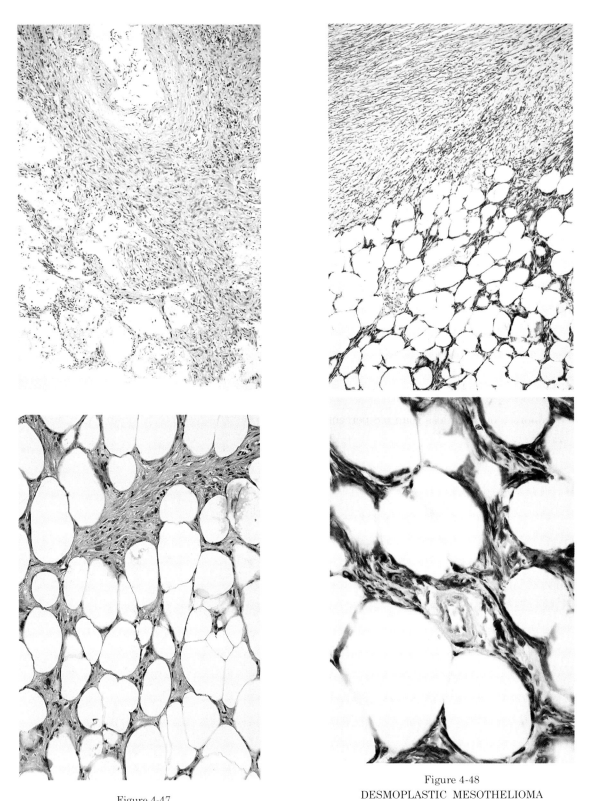

Figure 4-47
DESMOPLASTIC MESOTHELIOMA
Top: Invasion of alveolar septa.
Bottom: Invasion of adipose tissue.

Figure 4-48
DESMOPLASTIC MESOTHELIOMA
Top: Site of invasion of adipose tissue stained with a cocktail of monoclonal antibodies to low molecular weight keratins.
Bottom: Greater magnification of the invasive cells. A small artery serves as negative control for the immunostain.

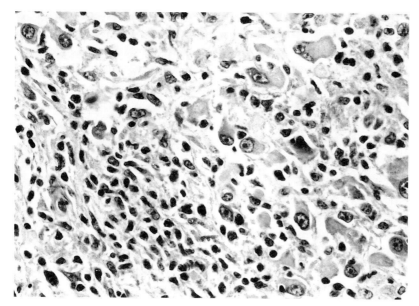

Figure 4-49
LYMPHOHISTIOCYTOID
MESOTHELIOMA
The tumor cells resemble histiocytes. There is a heavy infiltrate composed predominantly of small lymphocytes.

with finely divided chromatin, and nucleoli that are sometimes prominent. There is no evidence of tubulopapillary differentiation, but sarcomatoid spindle cell tumor may be observed in some areas. These tumors comprised less than 0.8 percent of 394 definite cases of DMM in the Australian Mesothelioma Surveillance Program (138).

Immunohistochemistry shows strong coexpression of cytokeratins and vimentin in the histiocyte-like cells, with no evidence of reactivity to leukocyte common antigen. Ultrastructural examination reveals a polymorphous population of fibrohistiocytic cells admixed with lymphocytes and plasma cells. However, sporadic cells exhibit mesothelial characteristics in the form of sinuous villiform processes, intracytoplasmic neolumina lined by microvilli, and intermediate filaments which tend to aggregate into tonofilament bundles (68). There is no evidence that the lymphohistiocytoid character of these tumors confers a prognostic advantage. Lymphohistiocytoid mesothelioma appears to represent one extreme of a spectrum of reactive lymphoplasmacytic infiltrates in predominantly sarcomatoid mesotheliomas (138).

Small Cell Mesothelioma. This tumor is characterized by a monotonous arrangement of uniform small cells with a high nuclear-cytoplasmic ratio (fig. 4-50). It superficially resembles small cell carcinoma and has been so misdiagnosed (187). When multiple specimen blocks from these tu-

mors are examined, regions of more typical DMM are seen. Small cell DMM does not show the streams, ribbons, rosettes, or hematoxyphilic blood vessels that characterize small cell carcinoma. However, in common with small cell carcinoma and other so-called neuroendocrine tumors, small cell DMM often expresses neuron-specific enolase (NSE) and sometimes stains with antibody Leu-7 (187,189). Nonsmall cell DMM also occasionally expresses NSE (189).

Mesothelioma In Situ. There is evidence supporting the concept of mesothelioma in situ of the pleura (327). In cases of this type, no pleural tumor masses are present but tiny dome-shaped nodules like "grains of sand" are seen, as are nodules ranging between 2 and 8 mm in size. Microscopically, the changes are characterized by a noninvasive surface mesothelial lesion composed of one or more layers of mesothelial cells demonstrating the cytologic characteristics of malignancy; the histologic pattern is of a flat monolayer or of papillary, tubular, or sheet-like arrangements (fig. 4-50). We have seen cases with what appeared to be extensive in situ mesothelioma, but on further sampling, microscopic areas of invasion were always seen. Nonetheless, the concept of mesothelioma in situ is a valuable one. Electron microscopy of the in situ component of a diffuse mesothelioma reveals preservation of the basal lamina (fig 4-51). Within a 0 to IV staging scheme, putative mesothelioma in situ would be stage 0.

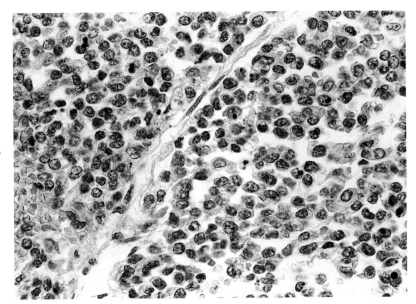

Figure 4-50
SMALL CELL MESOTHELIOMA
Small cells with high nuclear-cytoplasmic ratio.

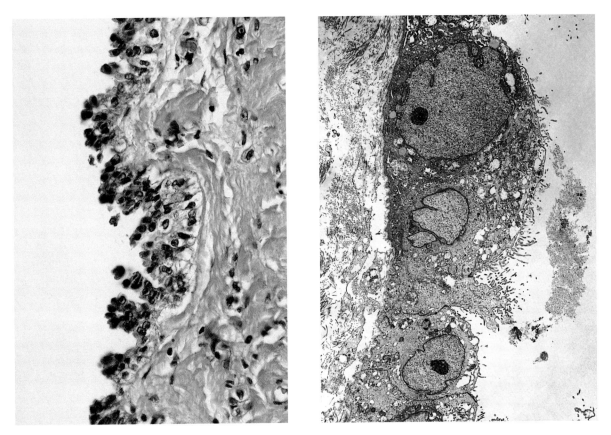

Figure 4-51
MALIGNANT MESOTHELIOMA IN SITU

A mesothelioma of the tunica vaginalis testis shows most of the much-distended tunica vaginalis covered by a single layer of highly atypical mesothelial cells with foci of micropapillary growth. Several small invasive foci were also found.

Left: Hematoxylin and eosin stain.

Right: Transmission electron micrograph. Note the typical surface microvilli, preservation of the basal lamina, and marked nuclear pleomorphism.

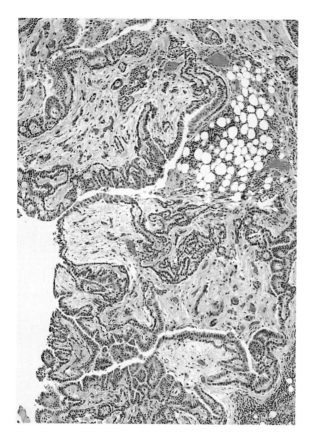

Figure 4-52
WELL-DIFFERENTIATED
PAPILLARY MESOTHELIOMA

Although the predominant pattern is papillary, some tubular structures are present.

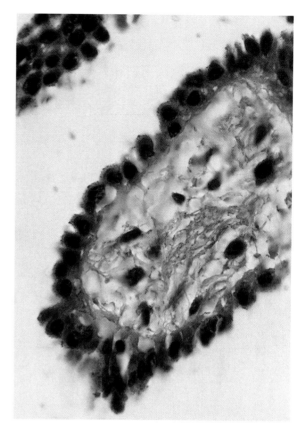

Figure 4-53
WELL-DIFFERENTIATED
PAPILLARY MESOTHELIOMA

Detail of a papilla showing a single layer of mesothelial cells with minimal atypia. Note brush borders correlating with presence of abundant microvilli.

Well-Differentiated Papillary Mesothelioma. This variant of mesothelioma usually occurs in the peritoneum and is most commonly seen in women, often in their 20s and 30s (81). Occasionally, well-differentiated papillary mesothelioma (WDPM) is found in other sites such as the tunica vaginalis testis (14), pericardium (121), and pleura (342). Although a few patients present with ascites or abdominal symptoms, the tumor is often found incidentally at laparotomy for some other indication. In a group of 22 patients with WDPM seen by one of the authors, 2 were sisters and 3 had possible exposure to asbestos (81).

Grossly, WDPM usually presents as multiple peritoneal nodules ranging from a few millimeters to several centimeters. The surfaces of the pelvic cavity, omentum, and mesentery are most often involved. Occasionally, small foci of tumor are present on the ovarian surface. In a few cases, only one

tumor nodule is seen (121). Satellite tumor nodules are occasionally seen microscopically (81).

Histologically, all WDPMs have a well-developed papillary architecture or tubulopapillary pattern in at least some areas (fig. 4-52). The papillae and tubules are lined by a single layer of uniform, cuboidal or flattened mesothelial cells with banal nuclear features (fig. 4-53). Mitoses are rare or absent. Occasionally the tumor cells are slightly more pleomorphic (fig. 4-54). Extensive fibrosis associated with irregularity of the glandular elements is common (fig. 4-55) and may be confused with malignant mesothelioma or adenocarcinoma. Psammoma bodies are present in some cases (fig. 4-56) (81).

The prognosis of WDPM is usually good (46). Nine of 10 untreated patients in the largest reported series (81) are alive and well at intervals between 1 and 14 years postoperatively. In another

49

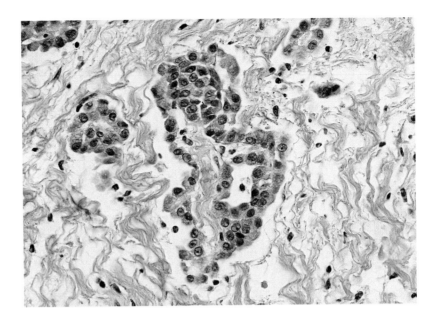

Figure 4-54
WELL-DIFFERENTIATED
PAPILLARY MESOTHELIOMA
Focus of moderate pleomorphism.

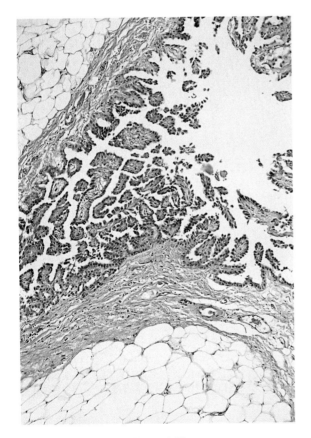

Figure 4-55
WELL-DIFFERENTIATED
PAPILLARY MESOTHELIOMA
Area of increased fibrosis.

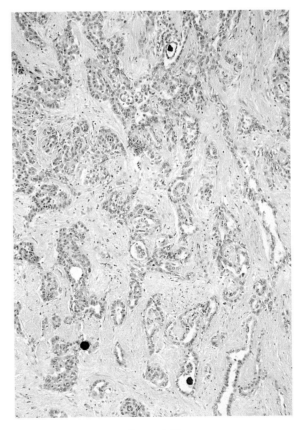

Figure 4-56
WELL-DIFFERENTIATED
PAPILLARY MESOTHELIOMA
Presence of psammoma bodies.

untreated patient, death occurred from carcinoma of the pancreas 29 years after the mesothelioma was originally diagnosed. Autopsy showed peritoneal nodules of similar microscopic appearance to those seen in the biopsy material 29 years earlier. In contrast, three of six female patients who received adjuvant therapy died. One of these patients was thought to have radiation enteritis. Another, who died 7 years after diagnosis, and had been treated intensively with radiation and chemotherapy, developed intestinal obstruction in the later stages of her illness.

Although WDPM appears to behave mainly in a benign fashion, the tumor occasionally may be more aggressive (81). A recent report describes a WDPM in a 51-year-old man who died 5 years after initial diagnosis of extensive peritoneal tumor, with resulting complete obliteration of the peritoneal cavity (46). The need for long-term follow-up is obvious. For now, the designation "well-differentiated" rather than "benign" seems appropriate; the term "borderline mesothelioma" has also been used (46). The available evidence justifies withholding adjuvant therapy in patients with WDPM unless there is a clear clinical indication that the tumor is progressing. Thus, the surgical pathology report should describe these tumors in terms that avoids their being treated as malignant mesothelioma.

When the lesions of WDPM are small, the differential diagnosis may include mesothelial hyperplasia. However, the striking papillary nature of many of these lesions and the absence of reactive changes in the adjacent serosa, antecedent disease, or previous surgery make hyperplasia improbable. Grossly, the peritoneal nodules may mimic peritoneal carcinomatosis. Microscopically, however, the uniformity of cells in WDPM (fig. 4-53), together with the absence of the nuclear features of malignancy, should readily distinguish it. Confusion with carcinoma is more likely in the small proportion of WDPMs in which there is some irregularity of the tubulopapillary elements associated with fibrosis (fig. 4-55). In such cases, examination of the nonfibrotic areas of the tumor should indicate the correct diagnosis. WDPMs are easily distinguished from primary or secondary borderline serous tumors involving the peritoneum by the absence of the stratified epithelium, cytologic atypia, and mitoses that are usually present in serous tumors. Another potential source of misdiagnosis

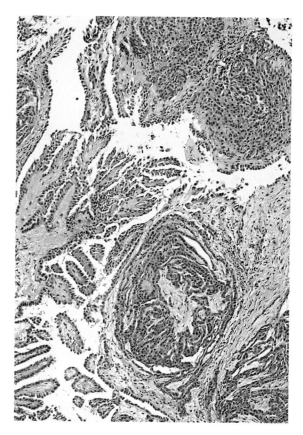

Figure 4-57
DIFFUSE MALIGNANT MESOTHELIOMA
OF THE PERITONEUM
Abundant papillary pattern which may be confused with well-differentiated papillary mesothelioma.

is the occasional case of peritoneal DMM in which coarse papillary elements, resembling those of WDPM, are prominent in parts of the tumor (fig. 4-57). However, the tumor masses of DMM are usually bulkier than those of WDPM and adequate histologic sampling shows obvious malignant features of DMM in other areas.

Malignant Mesothelioma of the Tunica Vaginalis Testis. These rare tumors are predominantly of the papillary type (fig. 4-58), but may have tubular or solid areas. The tumor cells sometimes have plentiful acidophilic cytoplasm and cytoplasmic vacuoles. Psammoma bodies are sometimes found. The clinical course is varied, and a separation into high- and low-grade malignant tumors has been suggested (127). A long asymptomatic interval from initial diagnosis to clinical recurrence has been noted (5), and spread to peritoneal surfaces as well as to inguinal and retroperitoneal

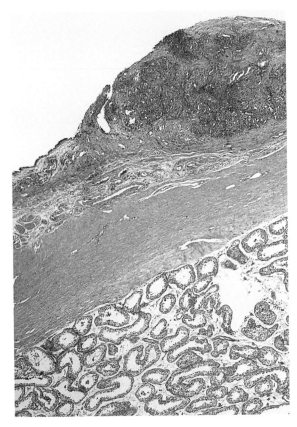

Figure 4-58
MALIGNANT MESOTHELIOMA OF THE
TUNICA VAGINALIS TESTIS

There is a nodule of mesothelioma with invasion of the underlying stroma.

lymph nodes may occur (313). Occasionally, malignant mesotheliomas have arisen from hernia sacs. Serous-surface papillary tumors of the tunica vaginalis have also been described (344). As the latter tumors arise from mesothelium, it is possible that, just as in the female pelvis (191), tumors that arise in the tunica vaginalis may have features intermediate between those of usual malignant mesothelioma and serous papillary tumor. The rare adenocarcinoma of the rete testis may be difficult to distinguish from mesothelioma if it has extended to involve the tunica vaginalis; a preponderance of growth in the testicular parenchyma helps to distinguish it (226). Benign fibrous tumors of possible mesothelial origin have been described in the scrotal sac (23).

Localized Malignant Mesothelioma. Most localized pleural neoplasms are benign and represent solitary fibrous tumors no longer regarded as true mesothelioma. Although very rare, localized forms of malignant mesothelioma that are histologically, ultrastructurally, and immunophenotypically indistinguishable from epithelial and biphasic forms of DMM have been reported (fig. 4-59) (74). In some of these cases there was a history of asbestos exposure, although no evidence of pleuropulmonary asbestosis was found. These tumors are aggressive, although complete surgical excision is curative in some cases.

Deciduoid Peritoneal Mesothelioma. Only three cases of this rare form of DMM have been reported (221,296). They affected young women and had an unusual histopathologic pattern closely resembling exuberant, ectopic decidual reaction of the peritoneum (fig. 4-60). In at least one case the appearance of the tumor led to an initial diagnosis of pseudotumoral deciduosis (296). The mesothelial origin of the tumor has been supported by ultrastructural and immunohistochemical findings (221,296). The tumor is highly malignant and is not correlated with asbestos exposure or endocrine imbalance.

Clinicopathologic Correlations. The most favorable prognostic factors at the time of diagnosis of DMM are absence of weight loss and absence of involvement of the visceral pleura (35).There is evidence that the clinical course may depend to some extent upon the histologic appearance. Patients with epithelial-type neoplasms survive significantly longer than do those with sarcomatous tumors; biphasic tumors occupy an intermediate position (35,84,98,126, 229,317). Within the epithelial group, tumors with abundant edematous or mucoid stroma have a better prognosis than the usual type of DMM (45). Epithelial DMM is associated with clinical features characteristic of carcinomas rather than sarcomas, including spread of tumor by direct extension, large pleural effusions, contralateral pleural effusions, ascites, metastases in regional lymph nodes, and, at times, response to radiotherapy. Sarcomatous DMM is associated with clinical features more characteristic of sarcomas, with frequent distant metastases, little or no effusion, and shorter survival times (111,172). With mixed tumors, having features of both carcinoma and sarcoma, large pleural effusions occur as frequently as with epithelial tumors, but survival is almost as poor as in sarcomatous cases. Prolonged survival has been reported in

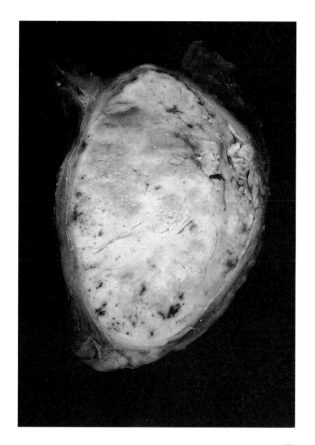 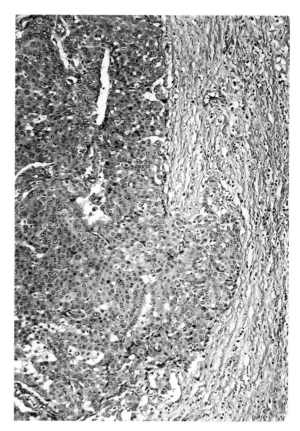

Figure 4-59
LOCALIZED MALIGNANT EPITHELIAL MESOTHELIOMA
Left: In this resected specimen, the tumor is sessile and the adjacent pleura normal.
Right: Photomicrograph of the same tumor showing a tubuloglandular pattern. (Figs. 3 and 4 from Crotty TB, et al. Localized malignant mesothelioma. A clinicopathologic and flow cytometric study. Am J Surg Pathol 1994;18:357–63.)

well-differentiated diffuse papillary mesothelioma of the peritoneum in women (81,106) and in occasional cases of desmoplastic mesothelioma (155). However, desmoplastic mesothelioma usually follows a rapid course, similar to that of sarcomatous mesothelioma (51). Female patients with limited disease, or those with symptoms for longer than 6 months before diagnosis, survive significantly longer than patients with more advanced disease at diagnosis (6,35, 84). A rare cystic form of mesothelioma (benign cystic mesothelioma) often behaves in an indolent fashion, with multiple pelvic operations required for control of recurrences (254,326). These variations must obviously be taken into account in assessment of therapy.

Cytology. Because most mesotheliomas present initially with an effusion in the affected cavity, examination of the aspirated fluid pres-

ents an opportunity for early and accurate diagnosis with minimum trauma and upset to the patient. However, the success rate in diagnosing mesothelioma from effusion fluid cytology has varied considerably and, in some populations, is very low (98). Recent reports indicate that, in experienced hands, reliable diagnosis of mesothelioma from effusion fluid is possible in 60 to 80 percent of mesotheliomas that are subsequently confirmed as such (272,329), and that false positives are rare. The importance of meticulous attention to technical detail has also been emphasized (329). At least three separate specimens should be examined when tumor is suspected but the initial cytologic examination is negative. Cell blocks should be made wherever possible, as these facilitate the application of special stains. Electron microscopy may be valuable (319). DNA ploidy analysis of pleural

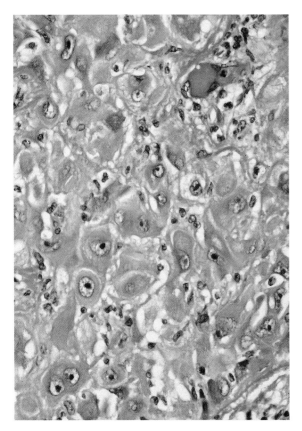

Figure 4-60
DECIDUOID MALIGNANT MESOTHELIOMA
Plump decidual-like mesothelial cells are seen. (Courtesy of Dr. A. Talerman, Philadelphia, PA.)

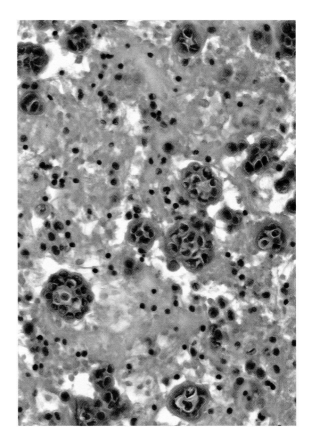

Figure 4-61
MALIGNANT PLEURAL MESOTHELIOMA
Cell block of pleural effusion showing formation of cell clusters (morulae). A dome-shaped protrusion of some of the cells at the periphery of the morula is seen.

mesotheliomas may be useful in diagnostically difficult cases in which histochemistry, immunohistochemistry, and electron microscopy have not provided an unequivocal distinction between adenocarcinoma and mesothelioma (102).

The cytologic diagnosis of mesothelioma is a two-stage process consisting of the demonstration of malignancy and the finding of mesothelial characteristics in the cancer cells. The criteria for malignancy include the usual nuclear changes of cancer, i.e., hyperchromasia, irregularity, enlargement, and nucleolar prominence. Because these changes are not always present or well developed, other morphologic pointers to malignancy should be sought. In epithelial mesothelioma, or mesothelioma with an epithelial component, the effusion is often cellular, and there may be considerable variation in the size of the malignant cells. Cell clusters or morulae

with a hobnail or scalloped contour are often seen in the effusion fluid (fig. 4-61). In approximately 50 percent of cases, there is a balanced mixture of mesothelioma cell clusters and single mesothelioma cells; in the remaining cases, either clusters or single cells predominate (272).

Mesothelial cells are identified by their cytoplasmic characteristics. Well-differentiated mesothelioma cells have abundant, optically dense cytoplasm, which usually stains more heavily than adenocarcinoma, and which often shows a fading-away or foamy appearance at the periphery. Signet ring cells are commonly seen in mesothelioma, due to the large cytoplasmic vacuoles with sharply defined margins. Lack of staining for epithelial mucin helps distinguish these vacuoles from those associated with adenocarcinoma. However, rare examples of mesothelioma that stain for neutral mucin have been

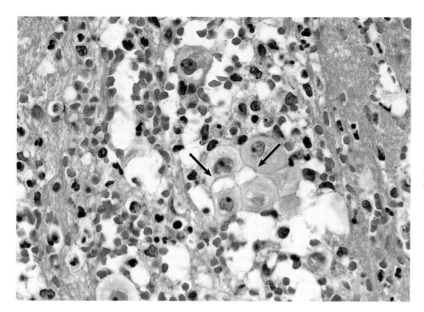

Figure 4-62
MALIGNANT PERITONEAL
MESOTHELIOMA
Cell block from the peritoneal fluid shows formation of "windows" at points of contact between tumor cells (arrows).

Figure 4-63
MALIGNANT EPITHELIAL
MESOTHELIOMA:
ULTRASTRUCTURAL
FEATURES

In this poorly differentiated epithelial mesothelioma, microvilli are scant and short (arrows), and desmosomes and tonofilaments are less prominent. Distinction from adenocarcinoma is not possible on ultrastructural grounds. (Courtesy of Dr. Douglas W. Henderson, Adelaide, Australia.)

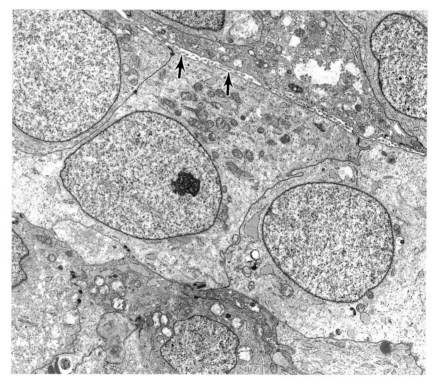

reported (180). Multinucleated giant cells are usually found without difficulty, and extensive cytomegaly is common (272). Opposing cell borders may show a gap or "window" between them (fig. 4-62), the result of an abundance of fine microvilli projecting from the opposing surfaces. Mesothelioma cells sometimes embrace or en-gulf each other. The nuclear-cytoplasmic ratio generally is almost normal (272). Large numbers of slender microvilli projecting from the surfaces of the tumor cells are seen ultrastructurally (figs. 4-63, 4-64). These abundant microvilli may be seen on conventional preparations as a "brush border," particularly in thin-sectioned cell blocks

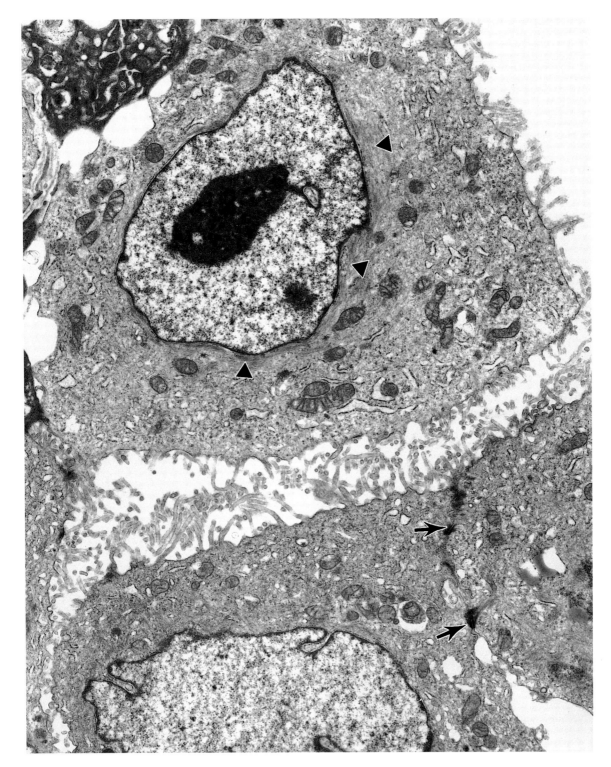

Figure 4-64

MALIGNANT EPITHELIAL MESOTHELIOMA: ULTRASTRUCTURAL FEATURES

Typical well-differentiated epithelial mesothelioma. Note the presence of abundant apical long sinuous surface microvilli. Gaps between cells are also microvilli-rich. Such gaps are responsible for the "windows" noticed in cytologic preparations. Well-developed desmosomes (arrows) and bundles of perinuclear tonofilaments (arrowheads) are abundant. (Courtesy of Dr. Douglas W. Henderson, Adelaide, Australia.)

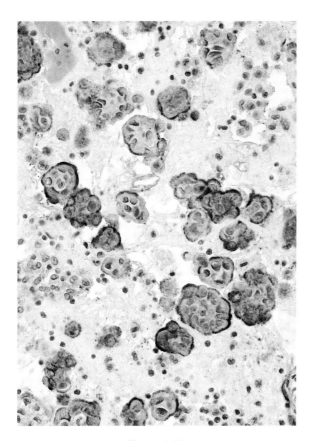

Figure 4-65
MALIGNANT MESOTHELIOMA OF THE PLEURA
Parallel section from the same case illustrated in figure 4-61 and stained with antibody HMFG-2. Note predominant membrane staining revealing a thick "brush border" type of pattern which correlates well with the presence of abundant long surface microvilli. A subsequent biopsy confirmed the diagnosis.

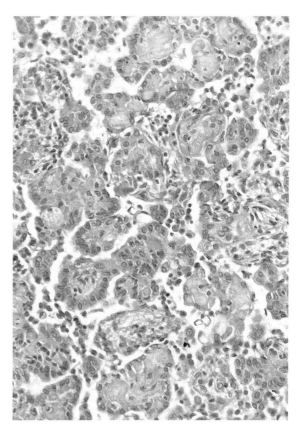

Figure 4-66
PAPILLARY MESOTHELIAL HYPERPLASIA
Cell block from a peritoneal effusion from a patient with benign hyperplasia of the peritoneal lining. It would be difficult to distinguish this cytologic preparation from one from a well-differentiated mesothelioma on routine cytologic examination.

or in cytospin preparations. Antibodies to various glycoproteins may facilitate the visualization of these structures (fig. 4-65). Although these findings help to identify the mesothelial origin of the cells, they do not differentiate neoplastic from reactive.

It is difficult to distinguish well-differentiated mesothelioma from reactive mesothelial hyperplasia (fig. 4-66). However, well-differentiated tumor cells are often accompanied by less well-differentiated transitional forms of the same population whose nuclear morphology indicates a malignant nature (fig. 4-67). Strong membrane staining for EMA or with antibody HMFG-2 is often seen in mesothelioma cells, but is unusual in reactive proliferations (19,329). Strong cytoplasmic staining with HMFG-2 is more common in adenocarcinoma than in mesothelioma (19). A monoclonal antibody

(MOC-31) to a 40-kd glycoprotein has been reported to immunoreact with all adenocarcinomas in serous fluids but not with reactive mesothelial or mesothelioma cells (257). Recent studies indicate that p53 protein accumulates in the nuclei in about 50 percent of mesotheliomas, but not in reactive mesothelial hyperplasia (fig. 4-68) (71,149,188,243). Nuclear immunostaining for this tumor suppressor protein helps distinguish well-differentiated mesothelioma cells from reactive mesothelial cells. We have seen weak to moderate immunostaining of occasional reactive mesothelial cells with antibodies to p53; thus, staining must affect a large proportion of the suspected cells to be diagnostically useful. Mesotheliomas have greater numbers of cells, larger cell clusters, and larger cell size than reactive hyperplasia (196). Adenocarcinoma metastatic to serous membranes

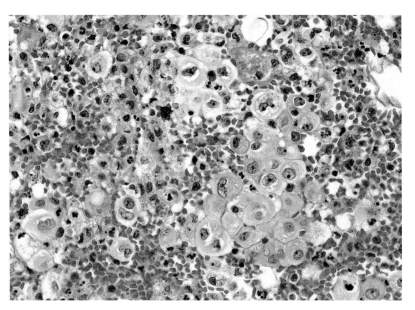

Figure 4-67
MALIGNANT PLEURAL
MESOTHELIOMA
Cell block showing atypical and typical
mesothelial cells.

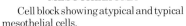

Figure 4-68
MALIGNANT PLEURAL
MESOTHELIOMA
Cell block stained with antibody
DO7 (Novocastra Laboratory, UK) to
p53 protein. Many of the neoplastic cells
show characteristic nuclear staining.

may be associated with prominent mesothelial cell hyperplasia (65,343), but unlike malignant mesothelioma, there is an absence of cells occupying an intermediate or transitional position between hyperplastic and malignant mesothelium. The percentage of cytologically positive cases, as well as the total number of such cases, is higher in the epithelial than in the sarcomatous form (297).

When the tumor cell type is undifferentiated or sarcomatous, distinction from other cancers is frequently impossible. The specific diagnosis must be based on other investigations such as immunocytochemistry and electron microscopy.

Blind needle biopsy is of some value in the detection of tumor and other disease processes involving the pleura, but it is less effective than cytology in the diagnosis of pleural cancers (110, 220). According to some studies, blind needle biopsy results in a higher proportion of correct diagnoses of mesothelioma than does cytology (98); others find that it rarely permits a definite diagnosis of mesothelioma (331). Our experience is that the small samples obtained do not allow

Table 4-8

DIFFERENTIAL DIAGNOSIS OF DIFFUSE MALIGNANT MESOTHELIOMA

Epithelial Mesothelioma
  Well differentiated
    Solid (epithelioid) or papillary mesothelial hyperplasia
  Moderately or poorly differentiated
    Tubulopapillary or tubular adenocarcinoma, epithelioid hemangioendothelioma
  Undifferentiated
    Poorly differentiated tumor, e.g., large and small cell carcinomas

Biphasic (Mixed) Mesothelioma
  Other biphasic tumors, e.g., synovial sarcoma, carcinosarcoma, epithelioid hemangioendothelioma
  Carcinoma with cellular stromal reaction
  Mesothelial hyperplasia with cellular serosal fibrosis
  Metaplasia of alveolar epithelium incorporated in the substance of tumors infiltrating lung, e.g., localized
    fibrous tumors of pleura

Sarcomatous Mesothelioma
  Sarcoma or spindle cell carcinoma arising in adjacent tissues
  Metastatic sarcoma
  Cellular serosal fibrosis

Desmoplastic Mesothelioma
  Reactive serosal fibrosis

---

a clear distinction between neoplasia and reactive hyperplasia or desmoplasia in many cases, and that, when obvious tumor is present, it is often difficult to distinguish DMM from metastatic carcinoma. However, biopsy findings have occasionally been positive when fluid cytology has been negative.

Frozen Section. We have seen numerous cases of mesothelioma in which frozen section examination was performed at the time of thoracotomy or laparotomy. Not infrequently, this has led to misdiagnosis or misclassification. Usually this has involved tubulopapillary epithelial mesothelioma being misdiagnosed as metastatic adenocarcinoma, or desmoplastic mesothelioma being identified as inflammatory fibrosis. Nonetheless, frozen section presents an invaluable opportunity to verify specimen quality and to select and prepare tissues adequately for immunohistochemistry and electron microscopy.

Differential Diagnosis. The main considerations in the differential diagnosis of mesothelioma are listed in Table 4-8. Peripheral adenocarcinomas of the lung may infiltrate the pleura extensively and are the best known gross and microscopic mimics of diffuse pleural mesothelioma of the tubular or tubulopapillary type ("pseudomesotheliomatous carcinoma") (87,135,

164). Histologically, it may be impossible to determine from routine sections whether a poorly differentiated glandular tumor is an adenocarcinoma or epithelial mesothelioma. Immunostaining for carcinoembryonic antigen (CEA), Leu-M1, B72.3, or other glycoprotein antigens and staining for neutral mucin can be helpful since most adenocarcinomas stain with more than one of these agents. Lack of staining supports a diagnosis of mesothelioma, although it does not exclude adenocarcinoma. The occurrence of unusual positive or negative reactions is discussed in the section on immunohistochemistry. Tumor cells with large cytoplasmic vacuoles that do not stain for mucin support a diagnosis of mesothelioma as does the ultrastructural presence of long or "bushy" microvilli, prominent desmosomal junctions, and tonofilaments. However, the absence of microvilli, tonofilaments, or desmosomes, or the presence of only short forms does not exclude poorly differentiated mesothelioma (76). Mucus granules or myelin figures, such as are found in some bronchioloalveolar carcinomas, are characteristic of adenocarcinomas. The presence of asbestos bodies or fibers in lung tissue, or asbestosis, does not provide any indication of the nature of the tumor, since inhalation of asbestos predisposes to both lung carcinoma and DMM.

Table 4-9

CHANGES ASSOCIATED WITH MESOTHELIAL HYPERPLASIA AND NEOPLASIA*

	Mesothelial Hyperplasia	Mesothelioma	Carcinoma
Grossly visible nodules	Uncommon	Common	Common
Papillary proliferation	Uncommon	Common	Sometimes
Slight to moderate cytologic atypia	Sometimes	Sometimes	Sometimes
Marked cytologic atypia	No	Common	Common
Necrosis of proliferating cells	No	Sometimes	Sometimes
Infiltration of adjacent tissue	Rare	Common	Common
Large cytoplasmic vacuoles	Usually inconspicuous	Often prominent	Usually inconspicuous
Lymphocytic infiltration	Sometimes	Sometimes	Sometimes
Epithelial membrane antigen	Negative or weak	Often strong, membrane pattern but no cytoplasmic staining	Often strong cytoplasmic staining
Nucleolar organizer regions	Low count	Higher count	—

*From reference 80.

Thymoma (141,236), thyroid carcinoma (208 , 210), soft tissue sarcomas (53,218,346), and renal cell carcinoma (195) are other tumors known to mimic DMM of pleura. Thymomas may involve the pleura diffusely and surround the lung (236). A well-developed biphasic histologic pattern strongly favors DMM over adenocarcinoma, but occasional pulmonary adenocarcinomas may be biphasic (47).

In the peritoneal cavity of women, differentiation of papillary mesothelioma from papillary serous carcinoma of the ovary may be difficult, especially when the state of the ovaries is uncertain. This problem is compounded by the existence of primary peritoneal tumors which show the same histologic features as papillary serous carcinoma of the ovary. In our experience, most diffuse papillary or tubulopapillary peritoneal tumors in women do not closely resemble, histologically, DMM of tubulopapillary epithelial type which occurs in the pleural cavity in both sexes (106). The presence of psammoma bodies, which are rare in mesotheliomas and common in papillary serous carcinomas; diastase-resistant PAS-positive material; and the immunohistochemical demonstration of several glycoprotein antigens supports the diagnosis of papillary serous carcinoma (Table 4-9). Tumors of intermediate histo-

logic appearance, as well as slowly progressing, well-differentiated, multifocal papillary mesotheliomas, may occur. In both sexes, metastatic gastrointestinal, breast, pancreatic, renal, and prostatic carcinomas have on occasion masqueraded very convincingly as peritoneal mesothelioma.

Certain spindle cell or anaplastic tumors of mesenchymal character arising in soft tissue or organs proximate to a serous membrane may be difficult to distinguish histologically from sarcomatous forms of DMM. Fibrosarcoma, leiomyosarcoma, rhabdomyosarcoma, malignant schwannoma, angiosarcoma, malignant fibrous histiocytoma, and synovial sarcoma have all been included in the differential diagnosis on occasion. However, unlike other tumors of sarcomatous appearance, sarcomatous DMM has the same gross characteristics regarding diffuse involvement of serous membrane as does usual DMM. In addition, sarcomatous DMM does not usually form a dominant mass such as is seen with many nonmesothelial sarcomas involving the lung or chest wall. Malignant fibrous histiocytoma is the most common soft tissue sarcoma involving the pleural cavity (218).

As previously discussed, the histologic appearance of mesothelial hyperplasia overlaps with that of epithelial DMM (Table 4-9). The degree of mesothelial proliferation and cytologic atypia, and the extent to which underlying tissues are infiltrated, are usually the most helpful histologic aids for distinguishing the two conditions in small biopsy specimens, but sometimes the evidence is inconclusive. Necrosis of mesothelial cells strongly favors DMM (193). Reactive proliferation of submesothelial fibroblasts appears similar to the fibrous areas of some diffuse sarcomatous or biphasic mesotheliomas. In these situations, the diagnostic problem can sometimes be resolved by an evaluation of the clinical and radiologic findings and careful assessment of the cytology of associated effusions. However, further direct sampling of the affected membrane may be required.

Ancillary Methods of Diagnosis. As already stated, it may be impossible to distinguish adenocarcinoma from epithelial mesothelioma with routine histologic stains, particularly when the tumor is poorly differentiated. Thus, ancillary diagnostic procedures are often required for enhancing diagnostic accuracy. Unfortunately, no currently available test is sufficient, by itself, to confirm the diagnosis of mesothelioma. Therefore, the accumulation of data obtained by several methods, coupled with the clinical findings, is often needed before a confident diagnosis can be made. It is recommended that all biopsy material should be handled in such a way as to optimize utilization of these ancillary procedures. Fixation in formaldehyde and electron microscopy fixative should be routine whenever the sample size permits. The tests that have been shown to be advantageous in the diagnosis of mesothelioma are histochemistry, assays of hyaluronate in tumor homogenates or in serous effusions, electron microscopy, and immunohistochemistry. Because each histologic type of mesothelioma has a different spectrum of differential diagnoses, the diagnostic value of these tests hinges in great part on the histologic type, as discussed in the following pages.

Histochemistry. *Glycosaminoglycans.* Normal mesothelial cells secrete glycosaminoglycans, particularly hyaluronate, which act as lubricants and facilitate the motion of the viscera within their respective cavities. Mesotheliomas, particularly well-differentiated ones, retain this secretory activity. If the material is appropriately fixed, many of the cytoplasmic vacuoles of well-differentiated epithelial mesothelioma may

be shown by histochemical methods to contain acid glycosaminoglycans. However, these methods are not sensitive enough, are difficult to reproduce, and often give false negative results because hyaluronic acid can leach out from the tissues when water-based fixatives, such as formalin, are used (324). In recent years, the histochemical demonstration of glycosaminoglycans has been largely replaced by immunohistochemical assays of several large molecular size glycoproteins, as discussed later. Since accumulation of cytoplasmic hyaluronate may be responsible for false positive histochemical and immunohistochemical stains in mesothelioma, tissue sections should be pretreated with hyaluronidase. Because many sarcomas also secrete glycosaminoglycans, the histochemical assay for these substances is of no value for distinguishing sarcomatous mesothelioma from sarcoma.

Mucins. Histochemical stains for neutral mucins, particularly the mucicarmine stain, help to distinguish epithelial DMM from adenocarcinoma but do not discriminate between sarcomatous mesothelioma and sarcoma. Although hyaluronidase-resistant cytoplasmic mucicarminophilia supports adenocarcinoma over mesothelioma, the test is relatively insensitive, particularly in poorly differentiated adenocarcinomas, which are often negative (24). PAS, after diastase digestion (dPAS), is less specific than the mucicarmine stain (24). Moreover, rare cases of bona fide, usually well-differentiated, mesothelioma displaying a few hyaluronidase-resistant mucicarmine-positive cytoplasmic vacuoles have been described (180). The above exceptions notwithstanding, in most instances the presence of hyaluronidase-resistant cytoplasmic mucicarminophilia strongly favors a diagnosis of adenocarcinoma over mesothelioma.

Electron Microscopy. The value of electron microscopy (EM) for separating epithelial mesothelioma from adenocarcinoma has been established by numerous studies (44,77,78,178,290,291, 321). However, EM is less effective for poorly differentiated epithelial DMM or for discriminating between sarcomatous mesothelioma and sarcoma.

The most useful ultrastructural finding in epithelial mesothelioma is the presence of long, thin, "bushy" and sinuous surface microvilli (figs. 4-63, 4-64), such as seen in non-neoplastic mesothelium (66,291,320,321). However, such microvilli may be

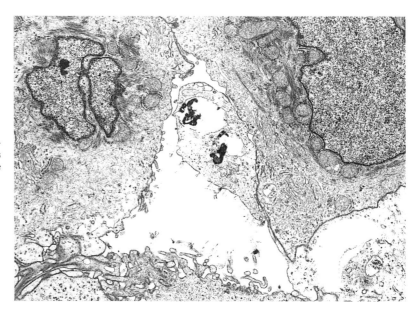

Figure 4-69
PSEUDOMESOTHELIOMATOUS
ADENOCARCINOMA
Electron micrograph from a peripheral adenocarcinoma of the lung that is invading the pleura. Microvilli are sparse and short.

very focal and difficult to find in less well-differentiated mesotheliomas, or only short microvilli, such as are often seen in adenocarcinoma, may be present (fig. 4-69). Poorly differentiated or sarcomatous mesothelioma may lack microvilli altogether as may adenocarcinoma. The microvilli of mesothelioma frequently involve large areas of the cell membrane and are often overlapping and branching, whereas in adenocarcinoma they tend to be restricted to the apical region of the tumor cells and are usually straight and nonbranching. Additionally, in well-fixed preparations of adenocarcinoma, particularly of gastrointestinal origin, the ultrastructural examination may reveal fine spikes of glycocalyx, core rootlets, and an underlying terminal web. These features are said not to be present in mesothelioma (fig. 4-69) (66).

It has been stated that the length/diameter ratio is the most useful diagnostic feature of the microvilli (321). A median length/diameter ratio of 11.90 in DMM and 5.28 in adenocarcinoma was reported by Burns et al. (44). Nonetheless, a gray zone exists, as these figures do overlap. For this reason, only a length/diameter ratio of 15 or above should be considered to be strongly supportive of epithelial DMM. Poorly differentiated epithelial DMM and sarcomatous DMM may lack microvilli, and electron microscopy is unlikely to be of value in these cases (76).

Other ultrastructural findings are of more doubtful significance. The presence of microvilli in direct contact with stromal collagen through defects in the basement membrane has been postulated to be specific of mesothelioma by some (88), but others report the same finding in adenocarcinoma (115). Abundant tonofilament bundles have been said to be characteristic of mesothelioma (321), whereas others find no difference in their numbers between mesothelioma and adenocarcinoma (25).

Immunohistochemistry. Numerous monoclonal antibodies (Mabs) to cell differentiation–related molecules have been established in recent years. Some of these are useful in the immunohistochemical diagnosis of mesothelioma. Although the literature reveals a fairly good agreement in results, some discrepancies exist. These are attributable in part to lack of standardization of tissue-processing and staining procedures, and in part to difficulty in avoiding case selection bias. Clearly, a study selecting only well-differentiated mesotheliomas and adenocarcinomas may yield more impressive results than does one that focuses on the more difficult to diagnose, less differentiated tumors. Such bias is difficult to avoid because of the absence of a "gold standard" for unambiguous identification of the less well-differentiated mesotheliomas.

Among the differentiation-related molecules useful in the diagnosis of mesothelioma are the

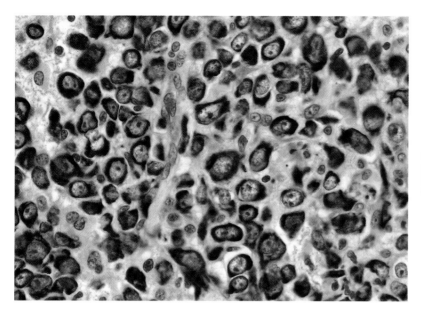

Figure 4-70
MALIGNANT MESOTHELIOMA
OF THE PLEURA
Section stained with a cocktail of monoclonal antibodies to cytokeratins. A ring-like distribution of the cytokeratin filaments, in close proximity to the nuclei, is observed in many of the cells.

intermediate filaments, particularly the cytokeratins, and a number of high molecular weight glycoproteins, referred to collectively as the "glycoproteins" in this text for convenience. Cytokeratins contribute to the distinction of sarcomatoid mesotheliomas, which nearly always express cytokeratins, from sarcomas, which usually do not.

As a general rule, the glycoproteins are commonly expressed by adenocarcinoma and infrequently by mesothelioma. Thus, the immunohistochemical diagnosis of mesothelioma is currently based on absence of staining with several antibodies to these glycoproteins. Admittedly, this is a less than satisfactory situation; it would be preferable to base the diagnosis on a positive result, rather than on a series of negative immunostains, by using a mesothelium (or mesothelioma)-specific antibody. Unfortunately, attempts to raise mesothelium-specific antibodies have been only partially successful to date.

Cytokeratins. Antibodies to intermediate filaments (IFs) are of great value in the immunohistochemical diagnosis of numerous neoplastic processes. The cytokeratins are the most diagnostically useful IFs. They are fairly specific markers of epithelial differentiation and maturation, and their expression is usually preserved in neoplastic cells. There are at least 20 individually gene-coded cytokeratins expressed in diverse combinations by various types of epithelia and their derived

tumors. Monoclonal antibodies with specificity restricted to most members of the cytokeratin family are now commercially available. Anomalous expression of cytokeratins by nonepithelial tumors is not common and is generally restricted to well-defined types. The IF phenotype of mesothelioma resembles that of normal and reactive mesothelial cells and is of diagnostic importance in specific circumstances.

The reliability of immunostains for IFs depends in great part on the quality of fixation. Moreover, in formalin-fixed specimens, some form of "epitope retrieval" procedure, such as protease digestion or boiling in citrate buffer, is obligatory for adequate results (124). Epitope retrieval may have to be fine tuned, depending on the duration of fixation (20). Some of the disagreements over results in the literature are due to lack of attention to these methodologic details. In our experience, with good immunohistochemical technique, virtually all mesotheliomas, as well as all adenocarcinomas, express low molecular weight cytokeratins (figs. 4-70–4-75) (60,63,315,316). It is apparent that the immunohistochemical demonstration of low molecular weight cytokeratins is of little value in distinguishing mesothelioma and adenocarcinoma (29,119,340). However, mesotheliomas may express more high molecular weight (epidermal) keratins than adenocarcinomas, and this feature may be diagnostically useful

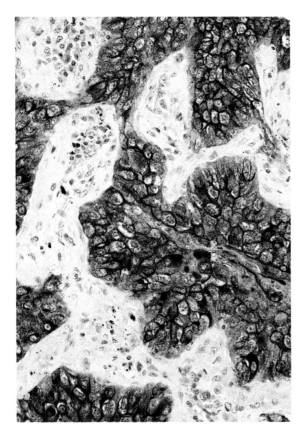

Figure 4-71
PSEUDOMESOTHELIOMATOUS ADENOCARCINOMA
Section from a peripheral lung adenocarcinoma with extensive pleural involvement, simulating mesothelioma. Perinuclear ring distribution is scant; the predominant pattern of distribution is at the cell periphery. (Stained with a monoclonal antibody cocktail to cytokeratins.)

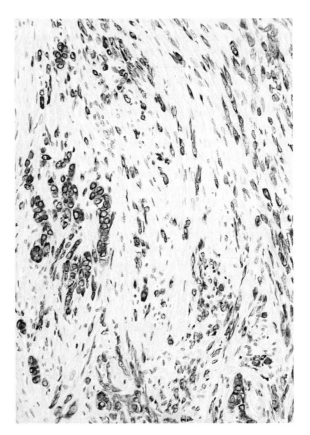

Figure 4-72
MALIGNANT MESOTHELIOMA
OF THE PLEURA
Biphasic pattern of growth is accentuated by the use of immunohistochemical staining for low molecular weight cytokeratins.

(30,213,340). Nonetheless, bona fide examples of adenocarcinoma, particularly those of lung origin, may also coexpress high and low molecular weight cytokeratins (233). Due to overlaps in the cytokeratin immunophenotype of mesothelioma and adenocarcinoma, cautious interpretation of the results of these immunostains is advised (222).

Useful differences in the pattern of distribution of cytokeratin filaments between mesothelioma and adenocarcinoma have been reported. A perinuclear array of filaments forming concentric rings is a common characteristic of mesothelioma (fig. 4-70), whereas in adenocarcinoma the staining tends to be more diffuse or predominantly below the cell membrane (fig. 4-71) (70,152). However, these differences are subtle, and the sections must be very thin and not overstained (152).

Broad-spectrum cytokeratin stains may confirm the biphasic nature of mesothelioma (fig. 4-72) or reveal the presence of minor biphasic components in a predominantly epithelial mesothelioma (fig. 4-74). It is important, however, not to misinterpret the presence of reactive submesothelial cytokeratin–containing spindle cells as evidence of a biphasic pattern (31). Such reactive cells are very common around foci of metastatic adenocarcinoma or mesothelioma near serosal surfaces (figs. 2-1, 4-74). They may be recognized by their bland cytologic features, as well as their distribution in parallel arrays close to the pleural surface. However, in metastatic carcinoma, when the tumor cells are very close to the serosal surface, a brisk proliferation of reactive mesothelial cells intimately intermixed with the tumor cells may be seen (fig. 4-74, right). In these cases, deposits of

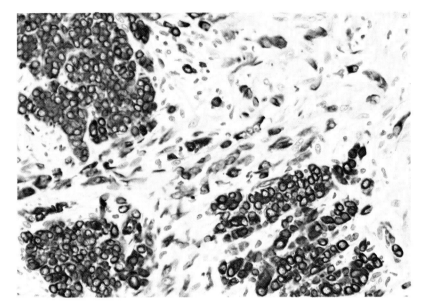

Figure 4-73
MALIGNANT MESOTHELIOMA
OF THE PLEURA
Minor biphasic component highlighted by immunohistochemical staining with a cocktail of monoclonal antibodies to low molecular weight cytokeratins.

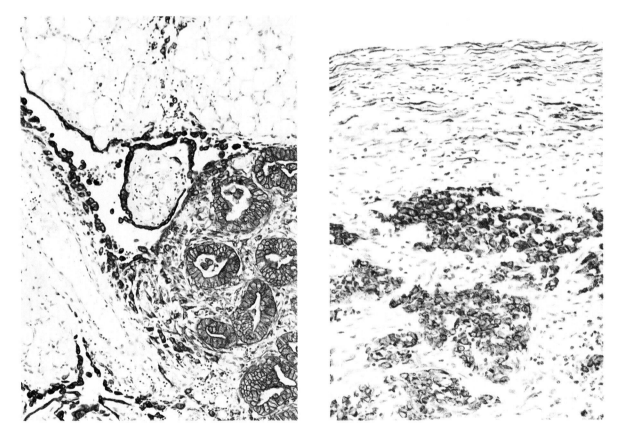

Figure 4-74
REACTIVE SUBMESOTHELIAL CELLS
Left: Cytokeratin immunostain of metastatic adenocarcinoma of the colon to the peritoneum. Reactive submesothelial spindle cells around the tumor cells are strongly stained. The tumor cells as well as the normal mesothelial surface cells are also stained.

Right: Cytokeratin immunostain of metastatic carcinoma to the pleura. Note the slender, fibroblast-like cells expressing keratins. Their long axes tend to be parallel to the pleural surface.

metastatic tumor away from the serosa will be devoid of such keratin-positive spindle cells in their stroma. In biphasic mesotheliomas, the number of keratin-positive spindle cells is not related to proximity to the serosal surface. Moreover, the spindle cells are oriented more randomly, have atypical cytologic features, and are often associated with a range of cells displaying features intermediate between epithelial and spindle cells.

The most important use of cytokeratins in the diagnosis of mesothelioma is for distinguishing sarcoma from sarcomatous mesothelioma. With good immunohistochemical technique virtually all sarcomatous mesotheliomas stain for low molecular weight cytokeratins, and the staining involves most of the cells (fig. 4-75). Conversely most nonmesothelial spindle cell sarcomas either do not express cytokeratins or do so only focally. Leiomyosarcoma and synovial sarcoma are the two spindle cell sarcomas most likely to express cytokeratins. Although these occasionally mimic mesothelioma clinically or grossly, they can readily be identified by their characteristic histologic appearance and distinct immunophenotypes (11,231,339).

Desmoplastic malignant mesothelioma, as previously discussed, presents a different diagnostic problem, since it may be mistaken for fibrous pleuritis or pleural scars, processes also known to involve cytokeratin-positive spindle cells (31,100). If the biopsy specimen is large enough to include normal lung or adipose tissue, the invasiveness of the cytokeratin-positive spindle cells in desmoplastic mesothelioma may be highlighted, whereas in reactive proliferations the submesothelial spindle cells tend to be sharply demarcated from the underlying tissues (figs. 2-1; 4-74, right). Additionally, in reactive lesions the cytokeratin-positive spindle cells are arranged in parallel (fig. 2-1; 4-74, right), whereas in desmoplastic mesothelioma they are arranged more haphazardly (fig. 4-48). Nonetheless, distinguishing between desmoplastic mesothelioma and reactive pleuritis can be extremely difficult, particularly when the biopsy specimens are small and fragmented (100); immunostains may not be of much assistance.

Spindle cell carcinoma metastatic to the pleura may infrequently enter the differential diagnosis of sarcomatous mesothelioma. Because cytokeratin stains are positive in both instances, they are not contributory. As already noted, mesotheliomas, including biphasic types, may contain

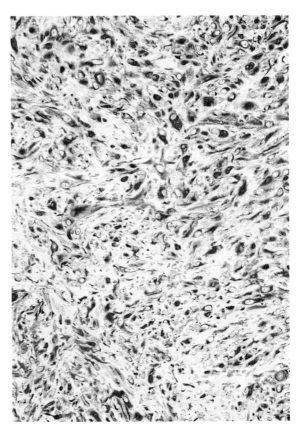

Figure 4-75

SARCOMATOUS MESOTHELIOMA OF THE PLEURA

This was stained with a cocktail of monoclonal antibodies to low molecular weight cytokeratins. Virtually every tumor cell expresses cytokeratins.

clear cells. Their presence may add to the difficulty in excluding a metastatic renal cell carcinoma with a sarcomatous component. The clinical picture, in particular the renal X rays or tomograms, may help to diagnose these cases.

Localized fibrous tumor of serous membranes (formerly called localized fibrous mesothelioma) should seldom be mistaken for sarcomatous or desmoplastic mesothelioma in view of its distinct gross and radiologic appearance. Also, the spindle cells of localized fibrous tumors of serous membranes are consistently cytokeratin negative (fig. 4-76), a feature that further helps to distinguish these two entities (2,86,100,258,283).

Thus, with rare exceptions, the expression of cytokeratins by the majority of the spindle cells in a pleural-based neoplasm should be interpreted as strongly supporting sarcomatous mesothelioma (49,214).

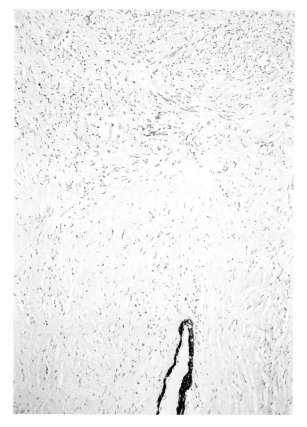

Figure 4-76
LOCALIZED FIBROUS TUMOR OF PLEURA
Cytokeratin stain showing absence of staining of the tumor cells. Strong staining of entrapped metaplastic epithelial cells of air-space origin serves as a positive control.

Vimentin. Vimentin is an IF expressed by most normal and neoplastic cells of mesenchymal origin. However, it may also be seen in normal epithelial cells and is also expressed by several types of tumors of epithelial origin (10). Consequently, earlier claims that the expression of vimentin by a pleural-based neoplasm favors mesothelioma over adenocarcinoma are no longer valid (145,230,332). Moreover, in our experience and that of others, epithelial mesothelioma may express scant or undetectable amounts of vimentin (230). Nonetheless, lung adenocarcinomas are seldom vimentin positive (215). Thus, coexpression of vimentin and cytokeratin by an epithelial-appearing pleural-based tumor should be considered to favor mesothelioma over pseudomesotheliomatous pulmonary adenocarcinoma. On the other hand, adenocarcinomas of the kidney, endometrium, and thyroid are frequent coexpressors of cyto-

keratin and vimentin, and any of these may present as pleural metastases (10). The pattern of cytoplasmic distribution of vimentin may be helpful in distinguishing adenocarcinoma from mesothelioma: in most vimentin-positive adenocarcinomas, vimentin predominates at the basal pole of the tumor cells, whereas in mesothelioma, the distribution tends to be more homogeneous within the cytoplasm (fig. 4-77).

Glycoproteins. As stated earlier, we apply the term glycoproteins to encompass a series of antibodies to epitopes of a diverse group of mucin-like glycoproteins. These antigens are more likely to be found in epithelium-derived tumors, particularly adenocarcinomas, than in mesotheliomas. For this reason, immunoreactivity of one or preferably more of these antibodies in a pleural-based tumor is generally regarded as supportive evidence for the diagnosis of adenocarcinoma. The expression of these glycoproteins varies depending on the degree of differentiation and site of origin of the adenocarcinoma. Therefore, a panel approach is currently employed so that the sensitivity of the assay is increased (270). Moreover, because bona fide mesothelioma may on occasion express one of these antibodies (and infrequently more than one), no diagnosis should be based on a single antibody. Finally, it must be emphasized that adenocarcinoma is not excluded even if the entire panel of antibodies to glycoproteins is negative, particularly when the biopsy specimen is scanty.

Although numerous antibodies have been proposed for differentiating mesothelioma and adenocarcinoma, the most commonly used are: carcinoembryonic antigen (CEA), Leu-M1 (CD15), B72.3, and Ber-EP4 (268–271). Less specific but at times very helpful are antibodies to milk fat globule–derived proteins such as HMFG-2. It is advisable to carefully titer each antibody to reduce nonspecific background staining, while at the same time maintaining maximum sensitivity. A panel of well-defined adenocarcinomas and mesotheliomas, preferably in a multitissue block (21), provides an economical control slide for this purpose.

Carcinoembryonic Antigen (CEA). Carcinoembryonic antigen is a member of a family of oncofetal glycoproteins originally isolated from extracts of colonic carcinoma (125). Studies have detected CEA in 70 to 100 percent of adenocarcinomas, but seldom in mesotheliomas (19,70,103,142,162,209, 233,240,268,269,304,315,318,330,332,337).

67

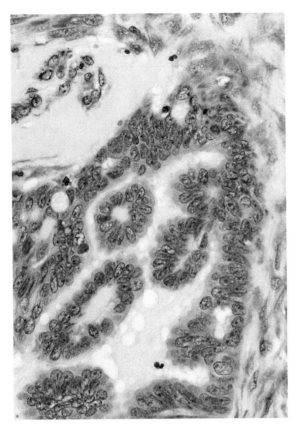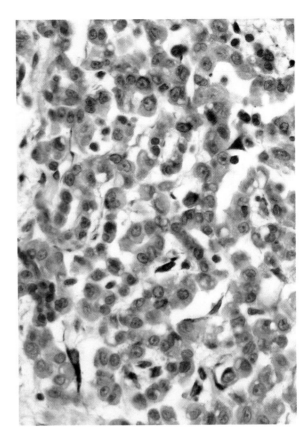

Figure 4-77
VIMENTIN IN MESOTHELIOMA AND ADENOCARCINOMA

Left: Pseudomesotheliomatous adenocarcinoma expressing vimentin. The filaments are predominantly arranged toward the basal pole of the tumor cells.

Right: Diffuse malignant mesothelioma of the pleura. Note the random distribution of the filaments which, in many cells, is perinuclear. (Both stained with monoclonal antibody V9 to vimentin.)

Many antibodies that immunoreact with different epitopes of CEA are currently available. Because of the complexity of the CEA family, the antibody chosen for diagnostic purposes may affect the results (85). Recently, the epitope reactivities of 52 Mabs against CEA from several laboratories were investigated by competitive inhibition. Five major epitope clusters, designated as Gold 1 to 5, were identified (133). Comparative immunohistologic studies in our laboratory have shown that antibodies that recognize epitopes of Gold groups 1 and 2 are the most sensitive for detecting CEA and have the least cross reactivity with normal tissues (101). The use of Mabs is recommended over antisera because the latter are usually broadly specific and may bind to members of the CEA family expressed by mesothelioma. Early reports of im-

munoreactivity of a large percentage of mesotheliomas for CEA were based on the use of antisera recognizing some of these less specific members of the CEA family, particularly the so-called nonspecific cross-reacting antigen (NCA) (240); it is useful to remember that some commercially available anti-CEA Mabs may bind to NCA and immunoreact with mesothelioma (85). Because NCA is abundant in neutrophils, such Mabs can readily be recognized by their immunoreactivity with leukocytes (19,268).

By employing noncross-reacting Mabs to CEA, we have found that immunoreactivity for CEA is exceptional in mesothelioma, and staining, if present, is usually weak and focal (195,233). The incidence of CEA positivity in adenocarcinoma depends on the site of origin, the choice of anti-CEA antibody, and the sensitivity of the method

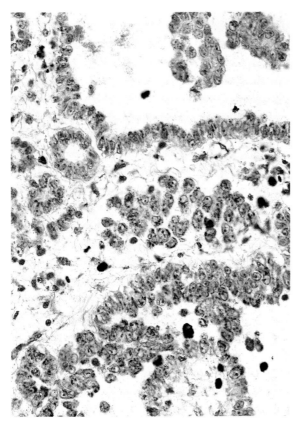

Figure 4-78
SPURIOUS STAINING OF MESOTHELIOMA
WITH CARCINOEMBRYONIC ANTIGEN ANTIBODIES
Example of a typical epithelial mesothelioma of the pleura showing coarse granular false positive reactivity with a monoclonal antibody to CEA. Several other monoclonal antibodies to different epitopes of CEA failed to reproduce this pattern of immunoreactivity, supporting its spurious nature.

employed. Adenocarcinomas of the lung and gastrointestinal tract are more likely to express CEA than are adenocarcinomas of other organs.

Some Mabs to CEA produce a coarse granular cytoplasmic staining in otherwise typical mesothelioma, as well as in non-neoplastic mesothelial cells, which should be considered to be spurious (fig. 4-78) (284). In contrast, most CEA-expressing adenocarcinomas exhibit a homogeneous, nongranular pattern. Also, some hyaluronate-rich mesotheliomas may show false positive staining for CEA. As stated earlier, these unwanted reactivities are eliminated by digestion of the tissue sections with hyaluronidase prior to immunostaining (248).

Leu-M1. Leu-M1 is one of a large group of antibodies against an antigen defined by the clus-

ter designation group 15 (CD15). These antibodies have in common their binding of a specific sugar sequence in the glycolipid lacto-N-fucopentaose III ceramide (8). This sugar sequence has also been referred to as X hapten or Lex. Initially, Leu-M1 was recognized as a myelomonocytic marker, also expressed by the neoplastic cells of Hodgkin's disease, macrophages, and leukocytes. Later, it was found to be expressed by many epithelial neoplasms and occasionally by mesothelioma (269). When positive, the pattern of staining is predominantly cytoplasmic and focal. The reported percentage of Leu-M1 positivity in adenocarcinoma has ranged from 60 to 100 percent (162,230,287,333, 337). Because Leu-M1 immunoreactivity is usually very focal, the likelihood of negative results in small biopsy specimens is increased. It is important to avoid areas of necrosis or of accumulation of neutrophils in the interpretation of Leu-M1–stained slides, because these areas may be difficult to interpret. Mesothelioma rarely immunoreacts with this Mab. However, as in the case of CEA, false positive staining may be found in hyaluronate-rich cases (248). Other antibodies that recognize the same sugar sequence as does Leu-M1 are also useful in differentiating mesothelioma and adenocarcinoma (174–176).

Ber-EP4. Ber-EP4 is a Mab raised using the breast cancer cell line MCF-7 as the immunogen. The antibody recognizes an epitope on the protein moiety of two glycopolypeptides that are present on a wide range of human epithelial cells and their tumors, and not in normal mesothelium (171). Typically, the lateral membranes of the cells of epithelium and epithelium-derived tumors stain with Ber-EP4, although some degree of cytoplasmic staining may be seen (fig. 4-79).

More than 85 percent of adenocarcinomas stain, often diffusely, with Ber-EP4, whereas only a rare mesothelioma stains, and only focally (211,271). However, some studies have reported a higher percentage of Ber-EP4–positive mesotheliomas than indicated earlier (113). Nevertheless, in these cases the staining was quite focal and weak. For these reasons the authors conclude that Ber-EP4 is a useful adjunct in the diagnosis of epithelial mesothelioma (113). Also, the broad distribution of the antigen in adenocarcinoma makes it useful in small biopsy samples or even for effusion fluids (168).

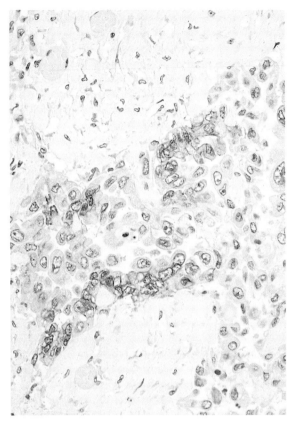

Figure 4-79
ADENOCARCINOMA METASTATIC
TO THE PLEURA

This tumor was stained with antibody BerEP4. Note the predominant membrane staining which involves lateral as well as apical membranes.

B72.3. Monoclonal antibody B72.3 is generated with a membrane-enriched fraction of human mammary carcinoma. It recognizes a high molecular weight glycoprotein called TAG-72 that is preferentially expressed by adenocarcinomas, and less often by non-neoplastic tissues. Thus, B72.3 is useful for distinguishing benign from malignant cells in histologic and cytologic preparations (146,147,163,179,223,295,301), and for distinguishing mesothelioma and adenocarcinoma (162,165,230,233,294,322,337). Most epithelial mesotheliomas do not stain for TAG-72; however, some show weak immunoreactivity with B72.3 in a small percentage of cells (less than 15 percent) (337). In any case in which the differential diagnosis is between adenocarcinoma and mesothelioma, strong immunoreactivity in more than 20 percent of the tumor cells with this Mab is strongly suggestive of adenocarcinoma.

Recent second generation Mabs that bind to different epitopes of the same or related molecules may be more suitable than B72.3 for immunohistochemistry (215).

Antibodies to Milk Fat Globules. Antisera and monoclonal antibodies have been raised against cell membranes isolated from milk fat globules. These antibodies recognize a heterogeneous group of high molecular weight glycoproteins. Several of the antibodies, some Mabs, some heterologous, have been directed to epithelial membrane antigen (EMA) and, as in the case of antibodies to CEA, they display variable immunoreactivities (275,300).

One milk fat globule–derived Mab, designated as HMFG-2, was reported to be useful for distinguishing mesothelioma and reactive mesothelial cells in serous effusions from adenocarcinoma (21). Some, but not all, subsequent studies have confirmed these observations (117,182,273, 279,304,337). Some of the controversy about HMFG-2 may be explained by differences in the interpretation of the immunostains. Cytoplasmic staining is uncommon in mesothelioma and prominent in adenocarcinoma with this Mab (fig. 4-80). On the other hand, mesothelioma may show strong membranous patterns of staining, often with a thick brush border–like appearance, and little cytoplasmic staining (fig. 4-81). Adenocarcinomas show either no membrane staining or only a thin pattern, and this is virtually always accompanied by cytoplasmic staining. Careful titration and thin (5 μm or less) sections are important for evaluating these differences in immunostaining. We currently use the antibody HMFG-2 (Unipath, Dedham, MA) at 1:4000 dilution. Because clear separation of membrane versus cytoplasmic staining is necessary in the interpretation of stains with HMFG-2, studies involving intact cells, such as cytospins of effusion fluids, are not reliable. Other antibodies, such as EMA, may also be used to disclose the presence of the thick brush border–like membrane patterns in mesothelioma. This is true for other antibodies prepared using mesothelioma cells as immunogens in the search of a mesothelioma-specific marker.

Lectins and Blood Group Antigens. Lectins are natural glycoproteins that bind specifically to carbohydrate groups such as those present in blood group antigens. Some lectins have been found to bind preferentially to adenocarcinoma, and thus

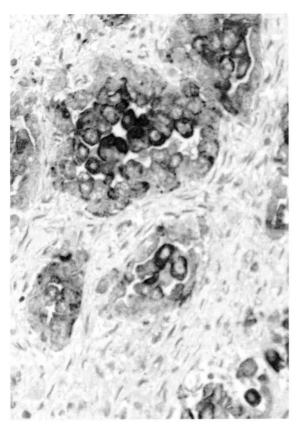

Figure 4-80
ADENOCARCINOMA METASTATIC
TO THE PLEURA
Note the predominantly cytoplasmic pattern of staining with antibody HMFG-2. The apical membranes are only slightly accentuated.

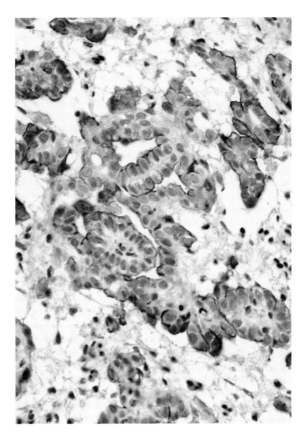

Figure 4-81
MALIGNANT EPITHELIAL
MESOTHELIOMA OF THE PLEURA
Note the predominantly thick membranous pattern of staining with antibody HMFG-2. The apical and free portions of the cell membrane are preferentially involved.

are useful in the distinction of adenocarcinoma from mesothelioma. Of the many lectins that have been tested, *Ulex europaeus* agglutinin (UEA) has been the most specific for this use (160,253).

Monoclonal antibodies with specificity for blood group antigens are now available and some of these, in particular those binding to Lewis blood group antigen, are capable of discriminating between mesothelioma and adenocarcinoma (148,227). In one study, 100 percent of adenocarcinomas showed diffuse, homogeneous membrane or cytoplasmic staining with Mabs to Lewis[y] and 78 percent with a Mab to Lewis[x]. Granular cytoplasmic staining was seen in about 20 percent of DMMs with these Mabs. However, this was considered not to be an impediment because the staining pattern was readily distinguished from the homogeneous pattern of immunoreactivity of adenocarcinoma (148).

We have tested a monoclonal antibody with specificity to Y blood group substance (type 2 chain), named BG-8 (Signet, Dedham, MA), for its capacity to distinguish mesothelioma from adenocarcinoma. At a high dilution (0.01 mg/ml), with the use of a standard ABC method on formalin-fixed, paraffin-embedded tumors, this antibody stained 10 of 100 epithelial or biphasic mesotheliomas and 108 of 125 adenocarcinomas (unpublished observations, H. Battifora, 1994). Additionally, the stains were stronger and more diffuse in the adenocarcinomas than in the few BG-8–positive mesotheliomas (fig. 4-82). We consider this to be another useful marker for distinguishing mesothelioma from adenocarcinoma and have added it to our routine diagnostic panel (Table 4-10). Several other antibodies, when used as a panel, may help to differentiate DMM from serous carcinomas (Table 4-11).

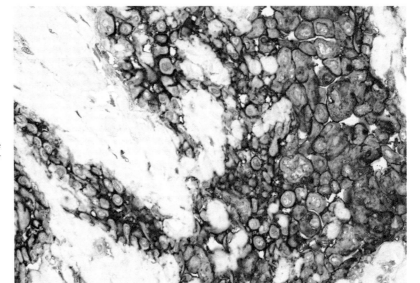

Figure 4-82
ADENOCARCINOMA METASTATIC
TO THE PLEURA
Note the strong and diffuse cytoplasmic staining with antibody BG-8 to Lewis[y] blood group antigen.

Table 4-10

MESOTHELIOMA ANTIBODY PANEL*

Antibody	Supplier **	Clone	Dilution[†]
Cytokeratins	Cocktail[‡]	[‡]	1:300
Vimentin (V9)	Dako	V9	1:100
Carcinoembryonic antigen	Boehringer Manheim	CJO65	1:5000
Leu-M1	Becton Dickinson	MMA	1:50
B72.3	Signet	B72.3	1:80
Ber-Ep4	Dako	Ber-EP4	1:400
BG8	Signet	F3	1:5000
HBME-1	Dako	HBME-1	1:5000
HMFG-2	Unipath	3.14.A3	1:4000

*Currently used by US-Canadian mesothelioma panel.
**Becton Dickinson, San Jose, CA; Boehringer Manheim, Indianapolis, IN; Dako, Carpenteria, CA; Unipath, Ogdensburg, NY; Signet, Dedham, MA.
[†]Dilution of antibody as supplied by manufacturer, for overnight incubation, ABC detection method. All slides are pretreated in microwave oven in citrate buffer solution before staining (126).
[‡]Cocktail of monoclonal antibodies to low molecular weight keratins AE1, Cam5.2, 35bH11, and UCD/PR 10/11 at optimal individual Mab titers.

Other Glycoprotein Antibodies. Many antibodies that bind preferentially to adenocarcinomas have been described (37,43,116,117,148,165, 235,273,293,294). It is likely that most of these antibodies recognize glycoproteins similar to those bound by the previously discussed glycoprotein antibodies.

Antimesothelial Antibodies. Clearly, it would be preferable to prepare antibodies to a mesothelium-specific antigen (if such an antigen exists), in order to base the diagnosis on positive immunoreactivity instead of a series of negative stains, as it is currently done. However, no true mesothelium-specific molecules have been identified

Table 4-11

IMMUNOHISTOCHEMISTRY OF PERITONEAL MESOTHELIOMA AND SEROUS CARCINOMAS*

Antigen	Mesothelioma (percent)	Serous Carcinoma (percent)
Cytokeratin	100	100
Epithelial membrane antigen	80	100
CA-125	15	90
Amylase	20	35
Leu-M1**	10	75
S-100 protein	10	85
Carcinoembryonic antigen	0	15
Placental alkaline phosphatase	0	65
B72.3	0	70
Vimentin	40	30
Human milk fat globule-2 (HMFG-2)	60	90

*From references 32a, 80, and 162.
**Extreme focal reactivity.

yet, although some antibodies showing partial specificity for mesothelial cells have been generated. One such molecule may be thrombomodulin. Collins et al. (67) reported that all of 31 mesotheliomas and only 4 of 48 (8 percent) adenocarcinomas stained with an antibody to thrombomodulin. However, others have not confirmed these findings (39).

An antiserum against a partially purified protein isolated from the cytoplasm of mesothelioma was prepared by Donna et al. (93,94) and was found to be capable of discriminating mesothelioma from adenocarcinoma on formalin-fixed, paraffin-embedded tissues. Several Mabs were prepared by Anderson et al. (4) who used a mesothelioma cell line as immunogen. One of the resulting Mabs, designated Mab 45, has shown partial specificity toward mesothelioma. Another Mab, named K1, was prepared against an ovarian tumor cell line as antigen source (57). This Mab has also shown partial specificity for mesothelioma and no reactivity with lung adenocarcinoma, but it may bind to adenocarcinomas arising from sites other than the lung. None of these antibodies is available commercially, and their diagnostic usefulness has not been

independently confirmed. A monoclonal antibody designated as ME1, generated from a mesothelial cell line, has been shown to be reactive with normal mesothelial cells and most mesotheliomas when studied in frozen sections (228). However, this antibody is not specific for mesothelial lineage since several adenocarcinomas immunoreact as well. Dr. Battifora, one author of this Fascicle, developed a Mab designated as HBME-1 using a suspension of cells from a well-differentiated epithelial mesothelioma as immunogen. As with other similar antibodies, HBME-1 is not entirely specific for mesothelial cells and a number of adenocarcinomas of various sites also immunoreact with it. However, in the context of an immunohistochemical/histochemical panel, the antibody can be quite useful. When a thick pattern of immunoreactivity of the cell surfaces, often including the intracytoplasmic lumina, is seen with HBME-1 and the rest of the diagnostic panel is negative, a diagnosis of mesothelioma is strongly supported. Moreover, comparative studies with electron microscopy (unpublished observations, H. Battifora, 1990) show an excellent correlation between the thick brush border pattern and the presence of abundant long microvilli. Additionally, in relatively well-differentiated mesotheliomas, Mab HBME-1 and comparable antimesothelial antibodies are more likely than the Mabs EMA or HMFG-2 to stain the thick membranes that are so useful diagnostically in histologic and cytologic preparations (fig. 4-83).

Tumor Suppressor Protein p53. Immunohistochemical assays of the tumor suppressor gene protein p53 have shown positivity in a large percentage of mesotheliomas, but not in reactive mesothelial proliferations (48,149,188,243). It is believed that immunostaining with antibodies to p53 protein indicate a point mutation in the gene leading to the production of a stabilized protein product. Thus, immunohistochemical assays for p53 may help to differentiate incipient forms of mesothelioma from reactive mesothelial proliferations (fig. 4-82). However, recent evidence suggests that caution may be necessary in the interpretation of these immunostains as other mechanisms may cause positive results (18,130). Because p53 abnormalities are common in many neoplastic processes, including many types of adenocarcinomas, this finding cannot be used for distinguishing mesothelioma from adenocarcinoma.

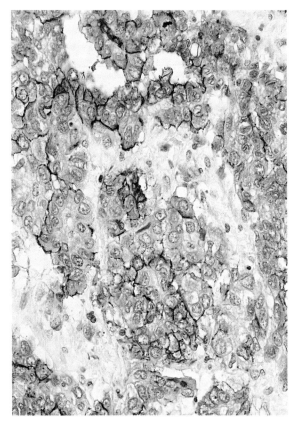

Figure 4-83
DIFFUSE MESOTHELIOMA, EPITHELIAL TYPE
This was stained with a monoclonal antibody raised against cell membrane preparations from mesothelioma cells in one of the authors' (H.B.) laboratory. The antibody highlights the thick brush border–like membrane on the tumor cells.

Immunohistochemical Mesothelioma Diagnostic Panel. Because of the insufficient specificity of the currently available antibodies used to distinguish mesothelioma from adenocarcinoma, a panel approach to immunodiagnosis is required. The distribution of the several glycoproteins detected by these antibodies varies depending, in part, on the origin of the adenocarcinoma. Because there is often no overlapping expression of these glycoproteins, the sensitivity of this diagnostic approach can be augmented by use of these antibodies concurrently, as a panel. The immunohistochemical panel presently used by the United States–Canadian Mesothelioma Panel is shown in Table 4-10. This panel only applies to differentiating epithelial mesothelioma from carcinoma. For purely sarcomatoid tumors, only cytokeratins and vimentin are used because the

rest of the antibodies are not contributory (218). However, additional antibodies may be necessary for further characterization of pleural-based sarcomas (49).

In our experience, if the mucicarmine stain is positive due to the presence of neutral mucin, several of the glycoprotein antibodies will be immunoreactive. Also, although it may appear paradoxical, mucicarmine positivity accompanied by lack of staining with all the glycoprotein antibodies listed in Table 4-10 should be interpreted as strongly favoring mesothelioma over adenocarcinoma. This is because abundant acid mucin is responsible for a false positive mucicarmine stain in most of these instances. Hyaluronidase treatment of the section prior to staining with mucicarmine results in a marked decrease or abrogation of the mucin staining in such cases.

It is important to remember that: 1) a rare mesothelioma may immunostain with one of the glycoprotein panel members; 2) such stains are usually quite focal and weak; 3) immunoreactivity with two or more antibodies, particularly if intense, should be interpreted as strongly favoring adenocarcinoma over mesothelioma; and 4) a negative result with all of the glycoproteins does not exclude the possibility of adenocarcinoma.

Flow Cytometry. Few studies evaluating the use of flow cytometry in the diagnosis and prognosis of mesothelioma are available. Three of these showed that a high percentage of mesotheliomas had a diploid or near-diploid DNA content, in contrast to other lung malignancies, particularly adenocarcinoma (42,96,242). However, the differences in DNA content between mesothelioma and adenocarcinoma, although statistically significant in one study (96), are not wide enough to warrant use of this method for diagnostic purposes. Another study compared the ploidy of mesothelial cell–rich benign effusions with that of mesothelioma (109). None of the effusions had abnormal DNA content, whereas 53 percent of 19 mesotheliomas were aneuploid. The investigators concluded that flow cytometry may be used for distinguishing reactive mesothelial proliferations from DMM in serous effusions. In two separate studies the possible prognostic value of flow cytometry in mesothelioma was explored (82,242). Both studies showed that patients whose mesotheliomas had a percentage of cells in S phase above the median (6 and 5.6 percent, respectively)

Table 4-12

ELEMENTS IN THE DIAGNOSIS OF DIFFUSE MESOTHELIOMA*

1. History and clinical features
2. Fluid cytology: cell histochemistry, immunohistochemistry, and fluid biochemistry as adjuncts
3. Studies excluding other sources of tumor, i.e., physical, radiographic, endoscopic
4. Gross morphology of the tumor: radiographic, endoscopic, exploratory surgery
5. Microscopic morphology of the tumor (needle or open biopsy): histochemistry, immunohistochemistry, and electron microscopy as adjuncts
6. Autopsy

*From reference 197.

had a lower overall survival than did those with S phases below the median. Ploidy, however, did not correlate with prognosis. Current data suggest that the usefulness of flow cytometry in the diagnosis and prognosis of DMM is limited.

Cytogenetics. Published reports on the cytogenetics of mesothelioma are scant. Hagemeijer et al. (129) studied 39 mesotheliomas by the direct method or after culture (or both). Nine cases showed a normal karyotype and 30 cases had complex and heterogeneous karyotypic abnormalities. However, two nonrandom abnormalities were detected: 1) loss of chromosomes 4 and 22 and chromosome arms 9p and 3p; and 2) gain of chromosomes 5, 7, and 20 with deletion or rearrangement of 3p in the few hyperdiploid cases in the series. Tiainien et al. (302) performed interphase cytogenetic studies by in situ hybridization (ISH), conventional karyotyping, and flow cytometry in 13 mesotheliomas. Both ISH and karyotyping revealed the same copy numbers for chromosomes 1 and 7 but ISH was more sensitive in detecting chromosomal aberrations. Despite the sparse data available thus far, it appears unlikely that cytogenetics will play an important diagnostic or prognostic role in the management of mesothelioma in the foreseeable future.

Hyaluronate Assays. Quantitative assay of hyaluronic acid (hyaluronate) in tumor tissue extracts or in serous effusions has been reported to be of value in distinguishing DMM from adenocarcinoma (159,184,219,324). High-performance liquid chromatography or radioassay are currently the preferred methods for this purpose (183). Although not without controversy (140), the majority of studies indicate that high levels of hyaluronate in serous effusions or in tumor homogenates are common in DMM and infrequent in adenocarcinoma. When dealing with tumor samples it is important to remember that hyaluronic acid leaches out from the specimen, if it is stored in aqueous solutions such as formalin. For that reason, any homogenate of a tumor or biopsy specimen prepared for hyaluronate assay must include the fixative to avoid false negative results (324).

Early Diagnosis. Information that contributes to a diagnosis of mesothelioma is listed in Table 4-12 in the chronological sequence in which it most logically becomes available. With increasing experience, more mesotheliomas can be precisely identified in the earlier stages, with consequent benefit to the patient in terms of therapeutic strategies and avoidance of unnecessary diagnostic or surgical procedures.

Because of the frequent development of cancer-related effusions, cytology plays a key role in the early detection of pleural and peritoneal cancer. In recent years, thoracoscopy and laparoscopy have increasingly supplemented cytology for early diagnosis. These procedures permit direct visualization of the cancerous process and increase the ability to take multiple biopsies. Most cases of pleural mesothelioma can be diagnosed after thoracotomy (36). In our experience, however, many biopsy procedures are still performed at thoracotomy or laparotomy, especially if DMM is being considered.

In recent years, immunohistochemical and ultrastructural studies have added greatly to the objective characterization of pleural tumors, especially DMM. Accurate diagnosis of mesothelioma is important for medicolegal reasons and because mesothelioma serves as a sentinel cancer in determining whether the concentrations of asbestos (and other mineral fibers) in the working or general environment have any carcinogenic potential.

Role of Autopsy. Although autopsy was essential for a definitive diagnosis of mesothelioma in the past, experience has shown that the tumor can often be accurately identified at an earlier stage based on its gross distribution, as defined by imaging techniques or surgery, and on its cytologic and histologic characteristics, based on immunohistochemistry and electron microscopy. Nonetheless, there are a small number of cases (about 5 to 10 percent in our experience) in which the diagnosis remains equivocal during the patient's life in spite of thorough investigation. In such instances only a carefully performed autopsy has the potential to resolve the diagnostic problem. Unfortunately, the massiveness and extent of the tumor at the time of death, the presence of secondary organ involvement, or an unusual microscopic appearance may still leave the issue in doubt.

The autopsy serves an additional important function in that it allows examination of the lungs for evidence of exposure to asbestos and asbestosis. This examination necessitates adequate sampling of lung tissue far from the tumor and its margins. Where special considerations (legal or research) justify the expense of electron microscopic studies, fiber counts, with identification of fiber types and the range of lengths of the fibers, may be carried out. It should be remembered that asbestosis is typically most pronounced at the bases of the lower lobes. The presence or absence of fibrous plaques on the parietal or diaphragmatic pleura should be noted, since this is also closely linked with exposure to asbestos and has been dubbed the "visiting" (or "calling") card of asbestos. Evidence based on these observations is of great epidemiologic importance and may be crucial in litigation.

The finding of asbestos fibers or bodies in the lungs is the hallmark of asbestos exposure. The bodies are usually 10 to 50 µm in length, but may be as long as 200 µm. They are usually 2 to 5 µm in diameter and have a varied morphology. Their varied appearances were described well in 1931 and are still valid (120). The most characteristic forms show a slightly fusiform structure with a knob at each end or a segmented rod with or without terminal bulbs. The bodies are golden yellow in unstained sections and brown in hematoxylin and eosin (H&E) preparations. They give a positive Prussian blue reaction, but are only weakly birefringent. It has been shown that all morphologically typical asbestos bodies consist of a central fiber which is coated by an iron-protein complex, and that the asbestos fiber is nearly always of the amphibole asbestos type (251). Nonasbestos substances (e.g., carbon, talc, mica) may form the core of ferruginous bodies, but these structures do not have the form of classic asbestos bodies and usually have black or yellow cores. However, erionite, a fibrous form of zeolite, can form ferruginous bodies that are indistinguishable from asbestos bodies by light microscopy (250).

The techniques used for demonstration of asbestos bodies vary greatly in sensitivity. Examination of H&E-stained 5-mm sections of lung is an insensitive method, and the finding of more than one asbestos body in a routine section usually indicates an occupational asbestos exposure. Iron-stained histologic sections are more sensitive than H&E, and usually show, in our experience, two to three times as many asbestos bodies as the corresponding H&E preparations. A much more sensitive technique involves digestion of wet lung tissue with sodium hypochlorite solution and collection of the dust residue on a membrane filter. This method has revealed asbestos bodies in 90 to 100 percent of routine autopsies from the general population (27,276), a finding that clearly reflects environmental exposure. With careful examination of iron-stained histologic sections of lung, asbestos bodies are unlikely to be found in a routine search if the asbestos body concentration in the tissue is less than 100 asbestos bodies/g wet lung. Because chrysotile appears to have little or no potential to form asbestos bodies, failure to find bodies has little significance as regards the extent of exposure to this most widely used form of asbestos. It should be recalled, however, that tremolite, an amphibole form of asbestos which often contaminates chrysotile ore, is a useful marker of exposure to chrysotile. Short chrysotile asbestos fibers tend to drift toward the pleura and have a particular tendency to accumulate in parietal pleura (173,260).

Asbestos fibers are much more numerous than asbestos bodies in the lung, and they are best seen by electron microscopy. Only 12 to 30 percent of the fibers found by electron microscopy are visible by phase contrast microscopy (9), and even lower percentages have been reported. Energy dispersive X ray spectrometry associated with transmission or scanning electron microscopy, or selected area electron diffraction transmission microscopy, permits typing of individual asbestos fibers (whether chrysotile, crocidolite, amosite, or other types of fiber) by their chemical and crystallographic properties. These techniques are of particular value in relation to epidemiologic studies and legal issues.

It has been claimed that the minimum pathologic findings that permit the diagnosis of asbestosis are the demonstration of fibrotic lesions in the walls of respiratory bronchioles and alveolar ducts, and the presence of asbestos bodies (72). However, others believe that the best evidence of early asbestosis is represented by interstitial fibrosis in the parenchyma surrounding the small airways, and that fibrosis of respiratory bronchioles and alveolar ducts is a separate and nonspecific reaction (59). Disagreement also persists as to how many asbestos bodies must be found, and their location, to permit asbestosis to be diagnosed. It has been stated that if even a single asbestos body is found in the lung tissue sections in the presence of diffuse interstitial fibrosis, the odds are good that one is dealing with asbestosis (59).

Mesothelioma Diagnostic Panels. In 1964, an International Union Against Cancer Working Group on Asbestos and Cancer suggested that national pathology reference panels for the diagnosis of mesothelioma be established (244). Within a few years, such panels were formed in several countries, including Great Britain, the United States, Canada, South Africa, and the Netherlands. Later, a mesothelioma panel of the Commission of European Communities was also established. Much of the material referred to these panels in their early years was related to epidemiologic studies, and, in order to increase diagnostic objectivity for this purpose, panels were asked to adopt the practice of grading individual tumors according to the degree of diagnostic certainty. Thus, terms such as "not a mesothelioma," "possible mesothelioma," "probable mesothelioma," and "definite mesothelioma" emerged. Grading was

often expressed in terms of a zero to four numerical system in which zero equaled "definitely not a mesothelioma" and four equaled "definite mesothelioma." Because it was unusual to achieve complete agreement among pathologists on a panel as to the diagnostic category to which a given tumor belonged, the majority opinion was effectively the working diagnosis. In reported epidemiologic studies, the expression of diagnostic certainty was sometimes further modified to such terms as "in favor" (of mesothelioma), "uncertain" or "against" (201) or "definite," "undecided," "insufficient histologic material," and "definitely not" (125).

The difficulty in achieving unanimity on the diagnosis and classification of many types of tumor is well known to pathologists. There is a subjective component in the histopathologic diagnosis of most tumors. This has been particularly evident for DMM because of the diversity of its microscopic appearance and the relative lack of specificity of some of the microscopic patterns seen in routine preparations. In one study, based on a collection of 27 representative slides, three experienced observers agreed on the diagnosis in only half of the cases (197). A further obstacle to consensus, in the authors' experience, has been the paucity of material and information sometimes given to panel pathologists. Although it has been observed that the availability of clinical and additional pathologic information changed pathologists' opinions little from those made on the basis of histology alone (201), the amount of such information, in our experience, has often been scanty. In reviews of United States and Canadian panel material in which the diagnosis of DMM had been suspected by the referring pathologist, an objective assessment was frequently seriously affected by deficiency in data or material for histologic examination (156,194). It has been emphasized that microscopic examination provides only one of a number of parameters which help diagnose DMM (157). Other parameters include gross morphology, histochemistry, immunohistochemistry, cytology of effusions, ultrastructural examination, radiologic and clinical findings, and exclusionary studies (Table 4-10). These parameters, singly or collectively, are frequently essential for a firm diagnosis of individual cases, especially in instances in which the microscopic material has a nonspecific appearance or is scanty (157).

Other factors may have prejudiced the objectivity of mesothelioma panel diagnoses: in one panel of nine pathologists, most of the cases were seen by only two members (197). It should also be realized that the criteria for the diagnosis of mesothelioma and its subtypes have often not been discussed in detail or agreed upon by panel members. For the most part, panel pathologists have made their diagnoses in isolation. There can be little doubt from other experience (241) that if panelists discussed problem cases with each other more often, there would be less difficulty in obtaining a consensus.

Despite its weaknesses, the panel system has almost certainly enhanced the overall quality of mesothelioma diagnosis as compared with the observations of individual experts. In recent years, the eight to ten members of a United States–Canadian mesothelioma panel reached a consensus of 75 percent or more on 70 percent of the referred material (195). Much of this material has been of a difficult or controversial nature. Panels have also provided continuing education for their members by informing the panelists how their opinions measure up to those of their colleagues and to the consensus, and by providing follow-up of patients. The availability of immunohistochemistry and electron microscopy has also contributed to the objectivity of the histopathologic diagnosis, especially in differentiating mesothelioma from metastatic adenocarcinoma (the most common differential diagnosis). It is also clear that performance will be improved further if the lessons learned from follow-up studies are applied critically.

Staging. The staging system proposed by Butchart in 1976 (Table 4-13) (45) is an easily applied tool for predicting survival and is thus the most commonly accepted system. Chahinian has recently modified this system by using the TNM staging system (Table 4-13) (55). Because absence of involvement of the visceral pleura is a favorable prognostic factor, it has been proposed that Butchart stage I be divided into stage IA (only parietal pleura involved) and stage IB (visceral pleura involved) (35). The most favorable prognostic factors are absence of weight loss at the time of diagnosis, absence of involvement of the visceral pleura (Butchart stage I), and epithelial histopathologic tumor type (35).

Table 4-13

SYSTEMS FOR CLINICOPATHOLOGIC STAGING OF DIFFUSE MALIGNANT MESOTHELIOMA OF PLEURA

Butchart Staging*
I.   Tumor confined to the ipsilateral pleura and lung
II. Tumor involving the chest wall, mediastinum, pericardium, contralateral pleura
III. Tumor involving both the thorax and abdomen or lymph nodes outside the chest
IV. Distant blood-borne metastases

Proposed TNM Staging**
 Primary tumor
   T1: Limited to ipsilateral pleura only
   T2: Superficial local invasion
   T3: Deep local invasion
   T4: Extensive direct invasion
 Lymph nodes (LN)
   N0: No positive LN
   N1: Positive ipsilateral hilar LN
   N2: Positive mediastinal LN
   N3: Positive contralateral hilar LN
 Metastases (M)
   M0: No M
   M1: Blood-borne or lymphatic M
 Stage
   I: T1N0M0
   II: T1+2, N0+1, M0
   III: T3, Nx†, M0 or T, N2+3
   IV: T4, Nx, M0+1

---

*Table 3 from reference 45.
**Table 1 from reference 54a.
†Any N.

Lymph node involvement also plays a significant prognostic role (288).

Treatment. This subject has been discussed in some detail in several recent reviews and reports (166,280,309). Treatment of DMM has proved disappointing, regardless of the modality used. Although it is doubtful that surgical resection could ever be curative because of the diffuse nature of the neoplastic process, there is some evidence that surgery may lengthen the survival period (7) and improve the quality of life (55). The most aggressive approach to pleural mesothelioma is radical extrapleural pneumonectomy, for which 3-year survival rates of 15 to 36 percent have recently been reported (309). However, only a small percentage of patients are candidates for this radical procedure. Radiotherapy appears to be ineffective in prolonging survival in cases of DMM of the pleura, but may have a useful role in palliation (12). However, it has been observed that radiotherapy may enhance invasion of the chest wall and the development of metastases (97). Chemotherapy offers the best prospect for treatment in most cases at the present time. Experience has been uneven, but there are reports of significant remissions with the use of adriamycin in multiple drug regimens (6,167,341), and a long duration of

response is occasionally reported (306). Chemotherapy with anthracyclines results in more remissions (9 of 21) than with nonanthracycline drugs (0 of 13) (280). The remission rate after primary chemotherapy with anthracyclines may be higher than for recurrent tumor (280). Particularly encouraging is the report that a considerable percentage of early stage I peritoneal DMMs may respond to chemotherapy, and that substantial palliation can be achieved by intensive combined treatment (7).

REFERENCES

1. Adamson IY, Bakowska J, Bowden DH. Mesothelial cell proliferation after instillation of long or short asbestos fibers into mouse lung. Am J Pathol 1993;142:1209–16.
2. Al-Izzi M, Thurlow NP, Corrin B. Pleural mesothelioma of connective tissue type, localized fibrous tumour of the pleura, and reactive submesothelial hyperplasia. An immunohistochemical comparison. J Pathol 1989;158:41–4.
3. Anderson HA, Lilis R, Daum SM, Fischbein AS, Selikoff IJ. Household-contact asbestos neoplastic risk. Ann NY Acad Sci 1976;271:311–23.
4. Anderson TM, Holmes EC, Kosaka CJ, Cheng L, Saxton RE. Monoclonal antibodies to human malignant mesothelioma. J Clin Immunol 1987;7:254–61.
5. Antman K, Cohen S, Dimitrov NV, Green M, Muggia F. Malignant mesothelioma of the tunica vaginalis testis. J Clin Oncol 1984;2:447–51.
6. _____, Blum RH, Greenberger JS, Flowerdew G, Skarin AT, Canellos GP. Multimodality therapy for malignant mesothelioma based on a study of natural history. Am J Med 1980;68:356–62.
7. _____, Osteen RT, Klegar KL, et al. Early peritoneal mesothelioma: a treatable malignancy. Lancet 1985;2:977–80.
8. Arber DA, Weiss LM. CD15: a review. App Immunohistochem 1993;1:17–30.
9. Ashcroft T, Heppleston AG. The optical and electron microscopic determination of pulmonary asbestos fibre concentration and its relation to the human pathological reaction. J Clin Pathol 1973;26:224–34.
10. Azumi N, Battifora H. The distribution of vimentin and keratin in epithelial and nonepithelial neoplasms. A comprehensive immunohistochemical study on formalin- and alcohol-fixed tumors. Am J Clin Pathol 1987;88:286–96.
11. _____, Ben-Ezra J, Battifora H. Immunophenotypic diagnosis of leiomyosarcomas and rhabdomyosarcomas with monoclonal antibodies to muscle-specific actin and desmin in formalin-fixed tissue. Modern Pathol 1988;1:469–74.
12. Ball DL, Cruickshank DG. The treatment of malignant mesothelioma of the pleura: review of a 5-year experience with special reference to radiotherapy. Am J Clin Oncol 1990;13:4–9.
13. Ball NJ, Urbanski SJ, Green FH, Kieser T. Pleural multicystic mesothelial proliferation: the so-called multicystic mesothelioma. Am J Surg Pathol 1990;14:375–88.
14. Barbera V, Rubino M. Papillary mesothelioma of the tunica vaginalis. Cancer 1957;10:183–9.
15. Baris I, Simonato L, Artvinli M, et al. Epidemiological and environmental evidence of the health effects of exposure to erionite fibres: a four-year study of the Cappadocian region of Turkey. Int J Cancer 1987;39:10–7.
16. _____, Artvinli M, Sahin AA. Environmental mesothelioma in Turkey. Ann NY Acad Sci 1979;330:423–32.
17. Battifora H. The pleura. In: Sternberg SS, ed. Diagnostic surgical pathology. New York: Raven Press, 1989:829–55.
18. _____. p53 immunohistochemistry. A word of caution [Editorial]. Hum Pathol 1994;25:435–7.
19. _____, Kopinski MT. Distinction of mesothelioma from adenocarcinoma. An immunohistochemical approach. Cancer 1985;55:1679–85.
20. _____, Kopinski MT. The influence of protease digestion and duration of fixation on the immunostaining of keratins. A comparison of formalin and ethanol fixation. J Histochem Cytochem 1986;34:1095–100.
21. _____, Mehta P. The checkerboard tissue block. An improved multitissue control block. Lab Invest 1990;63:722–4.
22. Beck B, Konetzke G, Ludwig V, Rthig W, Sturm W. Malignant pericardial mesotheliomas and asbestos exposure: a case report. Am J Ind Med 1982;3:149–59.
23. Benisch B, Peison B, Sobel NJ, Marquet E. Fibrous mesotheliomas (pseudofibroma) of the scrotal sac: a light and ultrastructural study. Cancer 1981;47:731–5.
24. Benjamin CJ, Ritchie AC. Histological staining for the diagnosis of mesothelioma. Am J Med Technol 1982;48:905–8.
25. Bewtra C, Greer KP. Ultrastructural studies of cells in body cavity effusions. Acta Cytol 1985;29:226–38.
26. Bégin R, Gauthier J, Desmeules M, Ostiguy G. Work-related mesothelioma in Quebec, 1967-1990. Am J Ind Med 1992;22:531–42.
27. Bhagavan BS, Koss LG. Secular trends in prevalence and concentration of pulmonary asbestos bodies—1940 to 1972. A necropsy study. Arch Pathol Lab Med 1976;100:539–41.

28. Bignon J, Sebastien P, Di Menza L, Payan H. French mesothelioma register. Ann NY Acad Sci 1979;330:455–66.

29. Blobel GA, Moll R, Franke WW, Kayser KW, Gould VE. The intermediate filament cytoskeleton of malignant mesotheliomas and its diagnostic significance. Am J Pathol 1985;121:235–47.

30. _____, Moll R, Franke WW, Vogt-Moykopf I. Cytokeratins in normal lung and lung carcinomas. I. Adenocarcinomas, squamous cell carcinomas and cultured cell lines. Virchows Arch [Cell Pathol] 1984;45:407–29.

31. Bolen JW, Hammar SP, McNutt MA. Reactive and neoplastic serosal tissue. A light-microscopic, ultrastructural, and immunocytochemical study. Am J Surg Pathol 1986;10:34–47.

32. _____, Thorning D. Mesotheliomas: a light-and electron-microscopical study concerning histogenetic relationships between the epithelial and the mesenchymal variants. Am J Surg Pathol 1980;4:451–64.

32a. Bollinger DJ, Wick MR, Dehner LP, et al. Peritoneal malignant mesothelioma versus serous papillary carcinoma. A histochemical and immunohistochemical comparison. Am J Surg Pathol 1989;13:659–70.

33. Bonser GM, Faulds JS, Stewart MJ. Occupational cancer of the urinary bladder in dyestuffs operatives and the lung in asbestos textile workers and iron-ore miners. Am J Clin Pathol 1955;25:126–34.

34. Boutin C, Rey F. Thoracoscopy in pleural malignant mesothelioma: a prospective study of 188 consecutive patients. Part 1: diagnosis. Cancer 1993;72:389–93.

35. _____, Rey F, Gouvernet J, Viallat JR, Astoul P, Ledoray V. Thoracoscopy in pleural malignant mesothelioma: a prospective study of 188 consecutive patients. Part 2: prognosis and staging. Cancer 1993;72:394–404.

36. _____, Viallat JR, Rey F. Thoracoscopy in diagnosis, prognosis and treatment of mesothelioma. In: Antman K, Aisner J, eds. Asbestos-related malignancy. Orlando: Grune & Stratton, 1987:301–22.

37. Bramwell ME, Ghosh AK, Smith WD, Wiseman G, Spriggs AI, Harris H. CA2 and CA3. New monoclonal antibodies evaluated as tumor markers in serous effusions. Cancer 1985;56:105–10.

38. Brooks JS, LiVolsi VA, Pietra GG. Mesothelial cell inclusions in mediastinal lymph nodes mimicking metastatic carcinoma. Am J Clin Pathol 1990;93:741–8.

39. Brown RW, Clark GM, Tandon AK, Allred DC. Multiple-marker immunohistochemical phenotypes distinguishing malignant pleural mesothelioma from pulmonary adenocarcinoma. Hum Pathol 1993;24:347–54.

40. Browne K. Is asbestos or asbestosis the cause of the increased risk of lung cancer in asbestos workers? [Editorial] Brit J Industr Med 1986;43:145–9.

41. _____, Smither WJ. Asbestos related mesothelioma: factors discriminating between pleural and peritoneal sites. Brit J Industr Med 1983;40:145–52.

42. Burmer GC, Rabinovitch PS, Kulander BG, Rusch V, McNutt MA. Flow cytometric analysis of malignant pleural mesotheliomas. Hum Pathol 1989;20:777–83.

43. Burnett RA, Deery AR, Adamson MR, Liddle C, Thomas M, Roberts GH. Evaluation of Ca1 antibody in pleural biopsy tissue. Lancet 1983;1:1158

44. Burns TR, Greenberg D, Mace ML, Johson EH. Ultrastructural diagnosis of epithelial malignant mesothelioma. Cancer 1985;56:2036–40.

45. Butchart EG, Ashcroft T, Barnsley WC, Olden MP. Pleuropneumonectomy in the management of diffuse malignant mesothelioma of the pleura. Experience with 29 patients. Thorax 1976;31:15–24.

46. Bürrig KF, Pfitzer P, Hort W. Well-differentiated papillary mesothelioma of the peritoneum: a borderline mesothelioma. Report of two cases and review of literature. Virchows Arch [A] 1990;417:443–447.

47. Cagle PT, Alpert LC, Carmona PA. Peripheral biphasic adenocarcinoma of the lung: light microscopic and immunohistochemical findings. Hum Pathol 1992;23:197–200.

48. _____, Brown RW, Lebovitz RM. p53 immunostaining in the differentiation of reactive processes from malignancy in pleural biopsy specimens. Hum Pathol 1994;25:443–8.

49. _____, Truong LD, Roggli VL, Greenberg SD. Immunohistochemical differentiation of sarcomatoid mesotheliomas from other spindle cell neoplasms. Am J Clin Pathol 1989;92:566–71.

50. Campbell GD, Greenberg SD. Pleural mesothelioma with calcified liver metastases. Chest 1981;79:229–30.

51. Cantin R, Al-Jabi M, McCaughey WT. Desmoplastic diffuse mesothelioma. Am J Surg Pathol 1982;6:215–22.

52. Carp NZ, Petersen RO, Kusiak JF, Greenberg RE. Malignant mesothelioma of the tunica vaginalis testis. J Urol 1990;144:1475–8.

53. Carter D, Otis CN. Three types of spindle cell tumors of the pleura. Fibroma, sarcoma and sarcomatoid mesothelioma. Am J Surg Pathol 1988;12:747–53.

54. Chabot JF, Beard D, Langlois AJ, Beard JW. Mesotheliomas of peritoneum, epicardium and pericardium induced by strain MC29 avian leukosis virus. Cancer Res 1970;30:1287–308.

54a. Chahinian AP. Malignant mesothelioma. In: Greenspan E, ed. Clinical interpretation and practice of cancer chemotherapy. New York: Raven Press, 1982:599–606.

55. _____, Holland JF. Treatment of diffuse malignant mesothelioma: a review. Mt Sinai J Med 1978;45:54–67.

56. _____, Pajak TF, Holland JF, Norton L, Ambinder RM, Mandel EM. Diffuse malignant mesothelioma. Prospective evaluation of 69 patients. Ann Int Med 1982;96:746–55.

57. Chang K, Pai LH, Pass H, et al. Monoclonal antibody K1 reacts with epithelial mesothelioma but not with lung adenocarcinoma. Am J Surg Pathol 1992;16:259–68.

58. Chovil A, Stewart C. Latency period for mesothelioma [Letter]. Lancet 1979;2:853.

59. Churg A. The diagnosis of asbestosis [Editorial]. Hum Pathol 1989;20:97–9.

60. _____. Immunohistochemical staining for vimentin and keratin in malignant mesothelioma. Am J Surg Pathol 1985;9:360–5.

60a. _____. Nonneoplastic diseases caused by asbestos. In: Churg A, Green FM, eds. Pathology of occupational lung disease. New York: Igaku-Shoin, 1988:220.

61. _____, Warnock ML, Bensch KG. Malignant mesothelioma arising after direct application of asbestos and fiberglass to the pericardium. Am Rev Respir Dis 1978;118:419–24.

62. _____, Wiggs B, Depaoli L, Kampe B, Stevens B. Lung asbestos content in chrysotile workers with mesothelioma. Am Rev Respir Dis 1984;130:1042–5.

63. Cibas ES, Corson JM, Pinkus GS. The distinction of adenocarcinoma from malignant mesothelioma in cell blocks of effusions: the role routine mucin histochemistry and immunohistochemical assessment of carcinoembryonic antigen, keratin proteins, epithelial membrane antigen, and milk fat globule-derived antigen. Hum Pathol 1987;18:67–74.

64. Cicala C, Pompetti F, Carbone M. SV40 induces mesotheliomas in hamsters. Am J Pathol 1993;142:1524–33.

65. Clement PB, Young RH. Florid mesothelial hyperplasia associated with ovarian tumors: a potential source of error in tumor diagnosis and staging. Int J Gynecol Pathol 1993;12:51–8.

66. Coleman M, Henderson DW, Mukherjee TM. The ultrastructural pathology of malignant pleural mesothelioma. Pathol Ann 1989;24:303–53.

67. Collins CL, Ordóñez NG, Schaefer R, et al. Thrombomodulin expression in malignant pleural mesothelioma and pulmonary adenocarcinoma. Am J Pathol 1992;141:827–33.

68. Constantopoulos SH, Theodoracopolous P, Dascalopoulos G, Saratlis N, Sideris K. Metsovo lung outside Metsovo. Endemic pleural calcifications in the ophiolite belts of Greece. Chest 1991;99:1158–61.

69. Cooper SP, Fraire AE, Buffler PA, Greenberg SD, Langston C. Epidemiological aspects of childhood mesothelioma. Pathol Immunopathol Res 1992;

70. Corson JM, Pinkus GS. Mesothelioma: profile of keratin proteins and carcinoembryonic antigen. Am J Pathol 1982;108:80–7.

71. Côté RJ, Jhanwar SC, Novick S, Pellicer A. Genetic alterations of the p53 gene are a feature of malignant mesotheliomas. Cancer Res 1991;51:5410–6.

72. Craighead JE, Abraham JL, Churg A, et al. The pathology of asbestos-associated disease of the lungs and pleural cavities: diagnostic criteria and proposed grading schema. Report of the Pneumoconiosis Committee of the College of American Pathologists and the National Institute for Occupational Safety and Health. Arch Pathol Lab Med 1982;106:544–96.

73. Cramer DW, Welch WR, Scully RE, Wojciechowski CA. Ovarian cancer and talc: a case-control study. Cancer 1982;50:372–6.

74. Crotty TB, Myers JL, Katzenstein AL, Tazelaar HD, Swensen SJ, Churg A. Localized malignant mesothelioma: a clinicopathologic and flow cytometric study. Am J Surg Pathol 1994;18:357–63.

75. d'Andiran G, Gabbiani GA. Metastasizing sarcoma of the pleura composed of myofibroblasts. In: Fenoglio CM, Woolf M, eds. Progress in surgical pathology. New York: Masson Publishing, 1980:34–40.

76. Dardick I, Al-Jabi M, McCaughey WT, Srigley JR, van Nostrand P, Ritchie AC. Ultrastructure of poorly differentiated diffuse epithelial mesotheliomas. Ultrastruct Pathol 1984;7:151–60.

77. _____, Al-Jabi M, McCaughey WT, Deodhare S, van Nostrand AW, Srigley JR. Diffuse epithelial mesothelioma: a review of the ultrastructural spectrum. Ultrastruct Pathol 1987;11:503–33

78. Davis JM. Ultrastructure of human mesotheliomas. JNCI 1974;52:1715–25.

79. Dawson A, Gibbs A, Browne K, Pooley F, Griffiths M. Familial mesothelioma: details of 17 cases with histopathologic findings and mineral analysis. Cancer 1992;70:1183–7.

80. _____, McCaughey WT. Pathology of the peritoneum: a review of selected topics. Sem Diag Pathol 1991;8:277–89.

81. Daya D, McCaughey WT. Well-differentiated papillary mesothelioma of the peritoneum. A clinicopathologic study of 22 cases. Cancer 1990;65:292–6.

82. Dazzi H, Thatcher N, Hasleton PS, Chatterjee AK, Lawson AM. DNA analysis by flow cytometry in malignant pleural mesothelioma: relationship to histology and survival. J Pathol 1990;162:51–5.

83. de Lajartre M, de Lajartre AY. Mesothelioma on the coast of Brittany, France. Ann NY Acad Sci 1979;330:323–32.

84. De Pangher Manzini V, Brollo A, Franceschi S, De Matthaeis M, Talamini R, Bianchi C. Prognostic factors of malignant mesothelioma of the pleura. Cancer 1993;72:410–7.

85. Dejmek A, Hjerpe A. Carcinoembryonic antigen-like reactivity in malignant mesothelioma: a comparison between different commercially available antibodies. Cancer 1994;73:464–9.

86. Dervan PA, Tobin B, O'Connor M. Solitary (localized) fibrous mesothelioma: evidence against mesothelial cell origin. Histopathology 1986;10:867–75.

87. Dessy E, Pietra GG. Pseudomesotheliomatous carcinoma of the lung. An immunohistochemical and ultrastructural study of three cases. Cancer 1991;68:1747–53.

88. Dewar A, Valente M, Ring NP, Corrin B. Pleural mesothelioma of epithelial type and pulmonary adenocarcinoma: an ultrastructural and cytochemical comparison. J Pathol 1987;152:309–16.

89. Doll R, Peto J. Effects on health of exposure to asbestos. In: Asbestos. London: Her Majesty Stationary Office, 1985.

90. _____, Peto J. Other asbestos-related neoplasms. In: Antman K, Aisner J, eds. Asbestos-related malignancy. Orlando: Grune & Stratton, 1993:81–98.

91. _____, Peto R. Quantitative estimates of avoidable risks of cancer in the United States today. In: The causes of cancer. Oxford: Oxford University Press, 1981:1243–5.

92. Doniach I, Swettenham KV, Hathorn MK. Prevalence of asbestos bodies in a necropsy series in east London: association with disease, occupation and domiciliary address. Br J Ind Med 1975;32:16–30.

93. Donna A, Betta PG. Differentiation towards cartilage and bone in a primary tumor of pleura. Further evidence in support of the concept of mesodermoma. Histopathology 1986;10:101–8.

94. _____, Betta PG, Bellingeri D, Marchesini A. New marker for mesothelioma: an immunoperoxidase study. J Clin Pathol 1986;39:961–8.

95. _____, Betta PG, Jones JS. Verification of the histologic diagnosis of malignant mesothelioma in relation to the binding of an antimesothelial cell antibody. Cancer 1989;63:1331–6.

96. El-Naggar AK, Ordez NG, Garnsey L, Batsakis JG. Epithelioid pleural mesotheliomas and pulmonary adenocarcinomas: a comparative DNA flow cytometric study. Hum Pathol 1991;22:972–8.

97. Elmes PC. Therapeutic openings in the treatment of mesothelioma. In: Bogovski P, Gillson JG, Timbrell V, Wagner JC, eds. Biological effects of asbestos. Lyon: International agency for research on cancer, 1973:277–82.

98. _____, Simpson JC. The clinical aspects of mesothelioma. Q J Med 1976;45:427–49.

99. Enterline PE. Asbestos and lung cancer. Attributability in the face of uncertainty. Chest 1980;78:377–9.

100. Epstein JI, Budin RE. Keratin and epithelial membrane antigen immunoreactivity in nonneoplastic fibrous pleural lesions: implications for the diagnosis of desmoplastic mesothelioma. Hum Pathol 1986;17:514–9.

101. Esteban JM, Paxton R, Mehta P, Battifora H, Shively JR. Sensitivity and specificity of gold types 1 to 5 anti-carcinoembryonic antigen monoclonal antibodies. Immunohistologic characterization in colorectal cancer and normal tissues. Hum Pathol 1993;24:322–8.

102. _____, Sheibani K. DNA ploidy analysis of pleural mesotheliomas: its usefulness for their distinction from lung adenocarcinomas. Modern Pathol 1992;5:626–30.

103. Faravelli B, D'Amore E, Nosenzo M, Betta PG, Donna A. Carcinoembryonic antigen in pleural effusions. Diagnostic value in malignant mesothelioma. Cancer 1984;53:1194–7.

104. Fishbein A, Suzuki Y, Selikoff IJ, Beckesi JG. Unexpected longevity of a patient with malignant pleural mesothelioma. Report of a case. Cancer 1978;42:1999–2004.

105. Fondimare A, Sebastien P, Monchaux G, Bignon J, Desbordes J, Bonnaud G. Variations topographiques des concentrations pulmonaires et pleurales en fibres d'amiante chez le sujets diversement exposs. Ann Anat Pathol (Paris) 1976;21:277–83.

106. Foyle A, Al-Jabi M, McCaughey WT. Papillary peritoneal tumors in women. Am J Surg Pathol 1981;5:241–9.

107. Fraire AE, Cooper S, Greenberg SD, Buffler P, Langston C. Mesothelioma of childhood. Cancer 1988;62:838–47.

108. Frank AL. Clinical observations following asbestos exposure. Environ Health Perspect 1980;34:27–36.

109. Frierson HF Jr, Mills SE, Legier JF. Flow cytometric analysis of ploidy in immunohistochemically confirmed samples of malignant epithelial mesothelioma. Am J Clin Pathol 1988;90:240–3.

110. Frist B, Kahan AV, Koss LG. Comparison of the diagnostic values of biopsies of the pleura and cytologic evaluation of pleural fluids. Am J Clin Pathol 1979;72:48–51.

111. Fusco V, Ardizzoni A, Merlo F, et al. Malignant pleural mesothelioma. Multivariate analysis of prognostic factors on 113 patients. Anticancer Res 1993;13:683–90.

112. Gaensler EA, Kaplan AI. Asbestos pleural effusion. Ann Int Med 1971;74:178–91.

113. Gaffey MJ, Mills SE, Swanson PE, Zarbo RJ, Shah AR, Wick MR. Immunoreactivity for BER-EP4 in adenocarcinomas, adenomatoid tumors, and malignant mesotheliomas. Am J Surg Pathol 1992;16:593–9.

114. Gerber MA. Asbestosis and neoplastic disorders of the hematopoietic system. Am J Clin Pathol 1970;53:204–8.

115. Ghadially FN, McCaughey WT, Perkins DG, Rippstein P. Diagnostic value of microvillus-matrix associations in tumors. J Submicrosc Cytol Pathol 1992;24:103–8.

116. Ghosh AK, Gatter KC, Dunnill MS, Mason DY. Immunohistological staining of reactive mesothelium, mesothelioma, and lung carcinoma with a panel of monoclonal antibodies. J Clin Pathol 1987;40:19–25.

117. _____, Mason DY, Spriggs AI. Immunocytochemical staining with monoclonal antibodies in cytologically negative serous effusions from patients with malignant disease. J Clin Pathol 1983;36:1150–3.

118. Gilks B, Hegedus C, Freeman H, Fratkin L, Churg A. Malignant peritoneal mesothelioma after remote abdominal radiation. Cancer 1988;61:2019–21.

119. Glass C, Kim KH, Fuchs E. Sequence and expression of a human type II mesothelial keratin. J Cell Biol 1985;101:2366–73.

120. Gloyne SR. The formation of the asbestosis body in the lung. Tubercle 1931;12:399–401.

121. Goepel JR. Benign papillary mesothelioma of peritoneum: a histological, histochemical and ultrastructural study of six cases. Histopathology 1981;5:21–30.

122. Goetz SP, Robinson RA, Landas SK. Extraskeletal myxoid chondrosarcoma of the pleura. Report of a case simulating mesothelioma. Am J Clin Pathol 1992;97:498–502.

123. Gold P, Freedman SO. Specific carcinoembryonic antigens of the human digestive system. J Exp Med 1965;122:467–81.

124. Gown AM, De Wever N, Battifora H. Microwave-based antigenic unmasking: a revolutionary new technique for routine immunohistochemistry. App Immunohistochem 1993;1:256–66.

125. Greenberg M, Davies TA. Mesothelioma register 1967-68. Br J Ind Med 1974;31:91–4.

126. Griffiths MH, Riddell RJ, Xipell JM. Malignant mesothelioma: a review of 35 cases with diagnosis and prognosis. Pathology 1980;12:591–603.

127. Grove A, Jensen ML, Donna A. Mesotheliomas of the tunica vaginalis testis and hernial sacs. Virchows Arch [A] 1989;415:283–92.

128. Grundy GW, Miller RW. Malignant mesothelioma in childhood. Report of 13 cases. Cancer 1972;30:1216–8.

129. Hagemeijer A, Versnel MA, Van Drunen E, et al. Cytogenetic analysis of malignant mesothelioma. Cancer Genet Cytogenet 1990;47:1–28.

130. Hall PA, Lane DP. p53 in tumour pathology: can we trust immunohistochemistry?—Revisited. J Pathol 1994;172:1–4.

131. Hammar SP, Bockus D, Remington F, Freidman S, LaZerte G. Familial mesothelioma: a report of two families. Hum Pathol 1989;20:107–12.

132. _____, Bolen JW. Pleural neoplasms. In: Dail DH, Hammar SP, eds. Pulmonary pathology. New York: Springer-Verlag, 1988:973–1028.

133. Hammarstrom S, Shively JE, Paxton RJ, et al. Antigenic sites in carcinoembryonic antigen. Cancer Res 1989;49:4852–8.

134. Hammond EC, Selikoff IJ, Churg J. Neoplasia among insulation workers in the United States with special reference to intra-abdominal neoplasia. Ann NY Acad Sci 1965;132:519–25.

135. Harwood TR, Gracey DR, Yokoo H. Pseudomesotheliomatous carcinoma of the lung. A variant of peripheral lung cancer. Am J Clin Pathol 1976;65:159–67.

136. Heller RM, Janower ML, Weber AL. The radiological manifestations of malignant pleural mesothelioma. Am J Roentgenol 1970;108:53–9.

137. Henderson DW, Attwood HD, Constance TJ, Shilkin KB, Steele RH. Lymphohistiocytoid mesothelioma: a rare lymphomatoid variant of predominantly sarcomatoid mesothelioma. Ultrastruct Pathol 1988;12:367–84.

138. _____, Shilkin KB, Whitaker D, et al. Unusual histological types and anatomic sites of mesothelioma. In: Henderson DW, Shilkin KB, Langlois SL, Whitaker D, eds. Malignant mesothelioma. New York: Hemisphere Publishing, 1992:140–63.

139. Higashihara M, Sunaga S, Tange T, Oohashi H, Kurokawa K. Increased secretion of interleukin-6 in malignant mesothelioma cells from a patient with marked thrombocytosis. Cancer 1992;70:2105–8.

140. Hillerdal G, Lindqvist U, Engtrm-Laurent A. Hyaluronan in pleural effusions and in serum. Cancer 1991;67:2410–4.

141. Hofmann W, Moller P, Manke HG, Otto HF. Thymoma. A clinicopathologic study of 98 cases with special reference to three unusual cases. Pathol Res Pract 1985;179:337–59.

142. Holden J, Churg A. Immunohistochemical staining for keratin and carcinoembryonic antigen in the diagnosis of malignant mesothelioma. Am J Surg Pathol 1984;8:277–9.

143. Hourihane D. A biopsy series of mesotheliomata, and attempts to identify asbestos within some of the tumors. Ann NY Acad Sci 1965;132:647–73.

144. Jara F, Takita H, Rao UN. Malignant mesothelioma of pleura: clinicopathologic observation. NY State J Med 1977;77:1885–8.

145. Jasani B, Edwards RE, Thomas ND, Gibbs AR. The use of vimentin antibodies in the diagnosis of malignant mesothelioma. Virchows Arch [A] 1985;406:441 8.

146. Johnston WW. Applications of monoclonal antibodies in clinical cytology as exemplified by studies with monoclonal antibody B72.3. The George N. Papanicolaou award lecture. Acta Cytol 1987;31:537–56.

147. _____, Szpak CA, Lottich SC, Thor A, Schlom J. Use of a monoclonal antibody (B72.3) as a novel immunohistochemical adjunct for the diagnosis of carcinomas in fine needle aspiration biopsy specimens. Hum Pathol 1986;17:501–13.

148. Jordon D, Jagirdar J, Kaneko M. Blood group antigens, Lewis^x and Lewis^y in the diagnostic discrimination of malignant mesothelioma versus adenocarcinoma. Am J Pathol 1989;135:931–7.

149. Kafiri G, Thomas DM, Shepherd NA, Krausz T, Lane DP, Hall PA. p53 expression is common in malignant mesothelioma. Histopathology 1992;21:331–4.

150. Kagan E, Jacobson RJ, Yeung K, Haidak DJ, Nachnani GH. Asbestos-associated neoplasms of B cell lineage. Am J Med 1979;67:325–30.

151. Kahn EI, Rohl A, Barrett EW, Suzuki Y. Primary pericardial mesothelioma following exposure to asbestos. Environ Res 1980;23:270–81.

152. Kahn HJ, Thorner PS, Yeger H, Bailey D, Baumal R. Distinct keratin patterns demonstrated by immunoperoxidase staining of adenocarcinomas, carcinoids, and mesotheliomas using polyclonal and monoclonal antikeratin antibodies. Am J Clin Pathol 1986;86:566–74.

153. Kannerstein M, Churg J. Desmoplastic diffuse malignant mesothelioma. In: Fenoglio CM, Wolff M, eds. New York: Progress in surgical pathology, Vol. II, 1980:19–29.

154. _____, Churg J. Peritoneal mesothelioma. Hum Pathol 1977;8:83–94

155. _____, Churg J, McCaughey WT. Asbestos and mesothelioma: a review. In: Sommers SC, Rosen PP, eds. Pathology annual Vol. 13, Part I. Philadelphia: WB Saunders Co, 1978:81–129.

156. _____, Churg J, McCaughey WT. Functions of mesothelioma panels. Ann NY Acad Sci 1979;330:433–9.

157. _____, McCaughey WT, Churg J, Selikoff IJ. Acritique of the criteria for the diagnosis of diffuse malignant mesothelioma. Mt Sinai J Med 1977;44:485–94.

158. Kauffman SL, Stout AP. Mesothelioma in children. Cancer 1964;17:539–44.

159. Kawai T, Suzuki M, Shinmei M, Maenaka Y, Kageyama K. Glycosaminoglycans in malignant diffuse mesothelioma. Cancer 1985;56:567–74.

160. Kawai T, Greenberg SD, Truong LD, Mattioli CA, Klima M, Titus JL. Differences in lectin binding of malignant pleural mesothelioma and adenocarcinoma of the lung. Am J Pathol 1989;130:401–10.

161. Keal EE. Asbestosis and abdominal neoplasms. Lancet 1960;2:1211–6.

162. Khoury N, Raju U, Crissman JD, Zarbo RJ, Greenawald KA. A comparative immunohistochemical study of peritoneal and ovarian serous tumors, and mesotheliomas. Hum Pathol 1990;21:811–9.

163. Kline TS, Lundy J, Lozowski M. Monoclonal antibody B72.3. An adjunct for evaluation of suspicious aspiration biopsy cytology from the breast. Cancer 1989;63:2253–6.

164. Koss M, Travis W, Moran C, Hochholzer L. Pseudomesotheliomatous adenocarcinoma: a reappraisal. Sem Diag Pathol 1992;9:117–23.

165. Koukoulis GK, Radosevich JA, Warren WH, Rosen ST, Gould VE. Immunohistochemical, analysis of pulmonary and pleural neoplasms with monoclonal antibodies B72.3 and CSLEX-1. Virchows Arch [Cell Pathol] 1990;58:427–33.

166. Krarup-Hansen A, Hansen HH. Chemotherapy in malignant mesothelioma: a review. Cancer Chemother Pharmacol 1991;28:319–30.

167. Kucuksu N, Thomas W, Ezdinli EZ. Chemotherapy of malignant diffuse mesothelioma. Cancer 1976; 37:1265–74.

168. Kuhlmann L, Berghäuser KH, Schäfer R. Distinction of mesothelioma from carcinoma in pleural effusions. An immunocytochemical study on routinely processed cytoblock preparations. Path Res Pract 1991;187:467–71.

169. Kwee WS, Veldhuizen RW, Golding RP, Donner R. Primary "adenosquamous" mesothelioma of the pleura. Virchows Arch [A] 1981;393:353–7.

170. Landrigan PJ. Preface. In: Landrigan PJ, Kazemi H, eds. The third wave of asbestos disease: exposure to asbestos in place. 643th ed. New York: New York Academy of Sciences, 1991:XV–XVI.

171. Latza U, Niedobitek G, Schwarting R, Nekarda H, Stein H. Ber-EP4: new monoclonal antibody which distinguishes epithelia from mesothelia. J Clin Pathol 1990;43:213–9.

172. Law MR, Hodson ME, Heard BE. Malignant mesothelioma of the pleura: the relation between histologic type and clinical behaviour. Thorax 1982;37:810–5.

173. LeBouffant L. Investigation and analysis of asbestos fibers and accompanying minerals in biological materials. Environ Health Perspect 1974;9:149–53.

174. Lee I, Radosevich JA, Chejfec G, et al. Malignant mesotheliomas. Improved differential diagnosis from lung adenocarcinomas using monoclonal antibodies 44-3A6 and 624A12. Am J Pathol 1986;123:497–507.

175. _____, Radosevich JA, Ma Y, Combs SG, Rosen ST, Gould VE. Immunohistochemical analysis of human pulmonary carcinomas using monoclonal antibody 44-3A6. Cancer Res 1985;45:5813–7.

176. _____, Warren WH, Gould VE, Radosevich JA, Ma Y, Rosen ST. Immunohistochemical demonstration of lacto-N-fucopentose III in lung carcinoma with monoclonal antibody 624A12. Path Res Pract 1987;182:40–7.

177. Legha SS, Muggia FM. Pleural mesotheliomas. Clinical features and therapeutic implications. Ann Intern Med 1977;87:613–21.

178. Lehto V, Virtanen I. Intermediate (10 nm) filaments in human malignant mesothelioma. Virchows Arch [Cell Pathol] 1978;28:229–34.

179. Lundy J, Lozowski M, Mishriki Y. Monoclonal antibody B72.3 as a diagnostic adjunct in fine needle aspirates of breast masses. Ann Surg 1986;203:399–402.

180. MacDougall DB, Wang SE, Zidar BL. Mucin-positive epithelial mesothelioma. Arch Pathol Lab Med 1992;116:874–80.

181. Mallory TB, ed. Case records of the Massachusetts General Hospital. Case 33111. N Engl J Med 1947;236:407–12.

182. Marshall RJ, Herbert A, Braye SG, Jones DB. Use of antibodies to carcinoembryonic antigen and human milk fat globule to distinguish carcinoma, mesothelioma and reactive mesothelium. J Clin Pathol 1984;37:1215–21.

183. Martensson G, Thylen A, Lindqvist U, Hjerpe A. The sensitivity of hyaluronan analysis of pleural fluid from patients with malignant mesothelioma and a comparison of different methods. Cancer 1994;73:1406–10.

184. Masse R, Sebastien P, Monchaux G, Bignon J. Experimental demonstration of the penetration of fibres into the gastrointestinal tract. In: Wagner JC, ed. Biologic effects of mineral fibres, Vol. 1. Lyon: IARC Sci Publ, 1980:321–8.

185. Matzel W, Schubert G. Hyaluronic acid in pleural fluids: an additional parameter for clinical diagnosis on diffuse mesotheliomas. Arch Geschwulstforsch 1979;49:146–54.

186. Maurer R, Egloff B. Malignant peritoneal mesothelioma after cholangiography with thorotrast. Cancer 1975;36:1381–5.

187. Mayall FG, Gibbs AR. The histology and immunohistochemistry of small cell mesothelioma. Histopathology 1992;20:47–51.

188. _____, Goddard H, Gibbs AR. p53 immunostaining in the distinction between benign and malignant mesothelial proliferations using formalin-fixed paraffin sections. J Pathol 1992;168:377–81.

189. _____, Jasani B, Gibbs AR. Immunohistochemical positivity for neuron-specific enolase and Leu-7 in malignant mesotheliomas. J Pathol 1991;165:325–8.

190. McAllister HA, Fenoglio JJ, Jr. Malignant tumors of the heart and pericardium. In: Hartmann WH, ed. Tumors of the cardiovascular system. Atlas of Tumor Pathology, 2nd Series, Fascicle 15. Washington: Armed Forces Institute of Pathology, 1978:77–8.

191. McCaughey WT. Papillary peritoneal neoplasms in females. Pathol Ann 1985;(Pt 2):385–404.

192. _____. Primary tumors of the pleura. J Pathol Bacteriol 1958;76:517–29.

193. _____, Al-Jabi M. Differentiation of serosal hyperplasia and neoplasia in biopsies. Pathol Ann 1986;21 (Pt 1):271–93.

194. _____, Al-Jabi M, Kannerstein M. A Canadian experience of the diagnosis of diffuse mesothelioma. In: Wagner JC, ed. Biological effects of mineral fibres, Vol. 1. Lyon: IARC Sci Publ 1980:207–10.

195. _____, Colby TV, Battifora H, et al. Diagnosis of diffuse malignant mesothelioma: experience of a U.S./Canadian Mesothelioma Panel. Modern Pathol 1991;4:342–53.

196. _____, Kannerstein M, Churg J. Tumors and pseudotumors of the serous membranes. Atlas of Tumor Pathology, 2nd Series, Fascicle 20. Washington, D.C.: Armed Forces Institute of Pathology, 1985.

197. _____, Oldham PD. Diffuse mesotheliomas: observer variation in histologic diagnosis. In: Bogovski P, Gilson JG, Timbrell V, Wagner JD, eds. Biological effects of asbestos. Lyon: IARC Sci Publ 1973:58–61.

198. _____, Wade OL, Elmes PC. Exposure to asbestos dust and diffuse pleural mesothelioma [Letter]. Br Med J 1962;2:1397.

199. McClure HM, Graham CE. Malignant uterine mesotheliomas in squirrel monkeys following diethylstilbestrol administration. Lab Anim Sci 1973;23:493–8.

200. McDonald AD, McDonald JC. Epidemiologic surveillance of mesothelioma in Canada. Can Med Assoc J 1973;109:359–62.

201. _____, McDonald JC. Epidemiology of malignant mesothelioma. In: Antman K, Aisner J, eds. Asbestos-related malignancy. Orlando: Grune & Stratton, 1987:31–55.

202. _____, McDonald JC. Malignant mesothelioma in North America. Cancer 1980;46:1650–6.

203. _____, McDonald JC, Pooley FD. Mineral fibre content of lung in mesothelial tumours in North America. Ann Occup Hyg 1982;26:417–22.

204. McDonald JC. Health implications of environmental exposure to asbestos. Environ Health Perspect 1985;62:319–28.

205. _____, Armstrong B, Case B, et al. Mesothelioma and asbestos fiber type. Evidence from lung tissue analyses. Cancer 1989;63:1544–7.

206. _____, McDonald AD. Epidemiology of mesothelioma from estimated incidence. Prev Med 1977;6:426–46.

207. Merewether ER. Annual report of the inspector of factories for the year 1947. London: His Majesty Stationary Office, 1949:79–81.

208. Merino MJ, Kennedy SM, Norton JA, Robbins J. Pleural involvement by metastatic thyroid carcinoma "tall cell variant": an unusual occurrence. Surg Pathol 1990;3:59–64.

209. Mezger J, Lamerz R, Permanetter W. Diagnostic significance of carcinoembryonic antigen in the differential diagnosis of malignant mesothelioma. J Thorac Cardiovasc Surg 1990;100:860–6.

210. Mizukami Y, Michigishi T, Nonomura A. Distant metastases in differentiated thyroid carcinomas: a clinical and pathological study. Hum Pathol 1990;21:283–90.

211. Moch H, Oberholzer M, Dalquen P, Wegmann W, Gudat F. Diagnostic tools for differentiating between pleural mesothelioma and lung adenocarcinoma in paraffin embedded tissue. Part I: immunohistochemical findings. Virchows Arch [A] 1993;423:19–27.

212. Moertel CG. Peritoneal mesothelioma. Gastroenterology 1972;63:346–50.

213. Moll R, Dhouailly D, Sun T. Expression of keratin 5 as a distinctive feature of epithelial and biphasic mesotheliomas. An immunohistochemical study using monoclonal antibody AE14. Virchows Arch [Cell Pathol] 1989;58:129–45.

214. Montag AG, Pinkus GS, Corson JM. Immunoreactivity for keratin proteins in sarcomatoid diffuse malignant mesothelioma: a diagnostic discriminant among malignant spindle cell tumors. Lab Invest 1985;52:44a.

215. Mullink H, Henzen-Logmans SC, Alons-van K, Kordelaar J, Tadema TM, Meijer CJ. Simultaneous immunoenzyme staining of vimentin and cytokeratins with monoclonal antibodies as an aid in the differential diagnosis of malignant mesothelioma from pulmonary adenocarcinoma. Virchows Arch [A] 1986;52:55–65.

216. Muraro R, Kuroki M, Wunderlich D, et al. Generation and characterization of B72.3 second generation monoclonal antibodies reactive with the tumor-associated glycoprotein 72 antigen. Cancer Res 1988;48:4588–96.

217. Musk AW, Dewar J, Shilkin KB, Whitaker D. Miliary spread of malignant pleural mesothelioma without a clinically identifiable pleural tumor. Aust NZ J Med 1991;21:460–2.

218. Myoui A, Aozasa K, Iuchi K, et al. Soft tissue sarcoma of the pleural cavity. Cancer 1991;68:1550–4.

219. Nakano T, Fujii J, Tamura S, et al. Glycosaminoglycan in malignant pleural mesothelioma. Cancer 1986;57:106–10.

220. Nance KV, Shermer RW, Askin FB. Diagnostic efficacy of pleural biopsy as compared with that of pleural fluid examination. Modern Pathol 1991;4:320–4.

221. Nascimento AG, Keeney GL, Fletcher CD. Deciduoid peritoneal mesothelioma. An unusual phenotype affecting young females. Am J Surg Pathol 1994;18:439–45.

222. Nelson WG, Battifora H, Santana H, Sun T. Specific keratins as molecular markers for neoplasms with a stratified epithelial origin. Cancer Res 1984;44:1600–3.

223. Ness MJ, Pour PM, Tempero MA, Linder J. Immunohistochemistry with monoclonal antibody B72.3 as an adjunct in the cytologic diagnosis of pancreatic carcinoma. Modern Pathol 1988;1:279–83.

224. Newhouse ML, Berry G. Predictions of mortality from mesothelial tumours in asbestos factory workers. Br J Ind Med 1976;33:147–51.

225. Nicholson CP, Donohue JH, Thompson GB, Lewis JE. A study of metastatic cancer found during inguinal hernia repair. Cancer 1992;69:3008–11.

226. Nochomowitz LE, Orenstein JM. Adenocarcinoma of the rete testis. Case report, ultrastructural observations, and clinicopathologic correlates. Am J Surg Pathol 1984;8:625–34.

227. Noguchi M, Nakajima T, Hirohashi S, Akiba T, Shimosato Y. Immunohistochemical distinction of malignant mesothelioma from pulmonary adenocarcinoma with anti-surfactant apoprotein, anti-Lewis[a], and anti-Tn antibodies. Hum Pathol 1989;20:53–7.

228. O'Hara CJ, Corson JM, Pinkus GS, Stahel RA. ME1. A monoclonal antibody that distinguishes epithelial-type malignant mesothelioma from pulmonary adenocarcinoma and extrapulmonary malignancies. Am J Pathol 1990;136:421–8.

229. Oels HC, Harrison EG Jr, Carr DT, Bernatz PE. Diffuse malignant mesothelioma of the pleura: a review of 37 cases. Chest 1971;60:564–70.

230. Ordóñez NG. The immunohistochemical diagnosis of mesothelioma. Am J Surg Pathol 1989;13:276–91.

231. _____, Mahfouz SM, Mackay B. Synovial sarcoma: an immunohistochemical and ultrastructural study. Hum Pathol 1990;21:733–49.

232. Osteen RT. Peritoneal mesothelioma. In: Antman K, Aisner J, eds. Asbestos-related malignancy. Orlando: Grune & Stratton, 1987:339–55.

233. Otis CN, Carter D, Cole S, Battifora H. Immunohistochemical evaluation of pleural mesothelioma and pulmonary adenocarcinoma. A bi-institutional study of 47 cases. Am J Surg Pathol 1987;11:445–56.

234. Owen WG. Mesothelial tumors and exposure to asbestos dust. Ann NY Acad Sci 1965;132:674–79.

235. Pallesen G, Jepsen FL, Hastrup J, Ipsen A, Hvidberg N. Experience with the Oxford tumour marker (Ca1) in serous effusions. Lancet 1983;1:132–6

236. Payne CB Jr, Morningstar WA, Chester EH. Thymoma of the pleura masquerading as diffuse mesothelioma. Am Rev Respir Dis 1966;94:441–6.

237. Perks WH, Crow JC, Green M. Mesothelioma associated with the syndrome of inappropriate secretion of antidiuretic hormone. Am Rev Respir Dis 1978;117:789–94.

238. Persaud V, Bateson EM, Bankay CD. Pleural mesothelioma associated with massive hepatic calcification and unusual metastases. Cancer 1970;26:920–8.

239. Peto J, Seidman H, Selikoff IJ. Mesothelioma mortality in asbestos workers: implications for models of carcinogenesis and risk assessment. Br J Cancer 1982;45:124–35.

240. Pfaltz M, Odermatt B, Christen B, Rutner J. Immunohistochemistry in the diagnosis of malignant mesothelioma. Virchows Arch [A] 1987;411:387–93.

241. Planteydt HT. Observer variation and reliability of the histopathological diagnosis of mesothelioma. Ann NY Acad Sci 1979;330:761–4.

242. Pyrhnen S, Laasonen A, Tammilehto L, et al. Diploid predominance and prognostic significance of S-phase cells in malignant mesothelioma. Eur J Cancer 1991;27:197–200.

243. Ramael M, Lemmens G, Eerdekens C, et al. Immunoreactivity for p53 protein in malignant mesothelioma and non-neoplastic mesothelium. J Pathol 1992;168:371–5.

244. Report and recommendations of the working group on asbestos and cancer: convened under the auspices of the Geographical Pathology Section of the International Union Against Cancer. Ann NY Acad Sci 1965;132:706–21.

245. Rich S, Presant CA, Meyer J, Stevens SC, Carr D. Human chorionic gonadotropin and malignant mesothelioma. Cancer 1979;43:1457–62.

246. Riddell RH, Goodman MJ, Moossa AR. Peritoneal malignant mesothelioma in a patient with recurrent peritonitis. Cancer 1981;48:134–9.

247. Risberg B, Nickels J, Wgermark J. Familial clustering of malignant mesothelioma. Cancer 1980;45:2422–7.

248. Robb JA. Mesothelioma versus adenocarcinoma: false positive CEA and Leu-M1 staining due to hyaluronic acid [Letter]. Hum Pathol 1989;20:400.

249. Roberts GH. Distant visceral metastases in pleural mesothelioma. Br J Dis Chest 1976;70:246–50.

250. Roggli VL. Asbestos bodies and nonasbestos ferruginous bodies. In: Roggli VL, Greenberg SK, Pratt PC, eds. Pathology of asbestos-associated diseases. Boston: Little Brown and Company, 1992:39–75.

250a._____, Coin P. Mineralogy of asbestos. In: Roggli VL, Greenberg SD, Pratt PC, eds. Pathology of asbestos-associated diseases. Boston: Little Brown & Co. 1992:1–18.

251. _____, McGavran MH, Subach J, Sybers HD, Greenberg SD. Pulmonary asbestos body counts and electron probe analysis of asbestos body cores in patients with mesothelioma: a study of 25 cases. Cancer 1982;50:2423–32.

252. Ros PR, Yuschok TJ, Buck JL, Shekitka KM, Kaude JV. Peritoneal mesothelioma. Radiologic appearances correlated with histology. Acta Radiol 1991;32:355–8.

253. Rosen-Levin E, Patil JR, Watson CW, Jagirdar J. Distinguishing benign from malignant pleural effusions by lectin immunocytochemistry. Acta Cytol 1989;33:499–504.

254. Ross MJ, Welch WR, Scully RE. Multilocular peritoneal inclusion cysts (so-called cystic mesothelioma). Cancer 1989;64:1336–46.

255. Ross R, Dworsky R, Nichols P, et al. Asbestos exposure and lymphomas of the gastrointestinal tract and oral cavity. Lancet 1982;2:1118–9.

256. Rubino GF, Scansetti G, Donna A, Palestro G. Epidemiology of pleural mesothelioma in north-western Italy (Piedmont). Br J Ind Med 1972;29:436–42.

257. Ruitenbeek T, Gouw AS, Poppema S. Immunocytology of body cavity fluids: MOC-31, a monoclonal antibody discriminating between mesothelial and epithelial cells. Arch Pathol Lab Med 1994;118:265–9.

258. Said JW, Nash G, Banks-Schlegel SP, Sassoon AF, Shintaku PI. Localized fibrous mesothelioma: an immunohistochemical and electron microscopic study. Hum Pathol 1984;15:440–3.

259. Sano ME, Weiss E, Gault ES. Pleural mesothelioma. Further evidence of its histogenesis. J Thorac Surg 1950;19:783–8.

260. Sebastien P, Janson X, Gaudichet A, Hirsch A, Bignon J. Asbestos retention in human respiratory tissues: comparative measurement in lung parenchyma and in parietal pleura. In: Wagner JC, ed. Biological effects of mineral fibers, Vol I. Lyon: IARC Sci Publ 1980:237–46.

261. Seidman H, Selikoff IJ, Hammond EC. Short term asbestos work exposure and long term observation. Ann NY Acad Sci 1979;330:61–87.

262. Selikoff IJ, Churg J, Hammond EC. Asbestos exposure and neoplasia. JAMA 1964;188:22–6.

263. _____, Hammond EC, Churg J. Asbestos exposure, smoking, and neoplasia. JAMA 1968;204:106–12.

264. _____, Hammond EC, Seidman H. Latency of asbestos disease among insulation workers in the United States and Canada. Cancer 1980;46:2736–40.

265. _____, Hammond EC, Seidman H. Mortality experience of insulation workers in the United States and Canada, 1943–1976. Ann NY Acad Sci 1979;330:91–116.

266. _____, Lee DH. Asbestos and disease. New York: Academic Press, 1978.

267. _____, Seidman H. Cancer of the pancreas among asbestos insulation workers. Cancer 1981;47:1469–73.

268. Sheibani K, Battifora H, Burke JS. Antigenic phenotype of malignant mesotheliomas and pulmonary adenocarcinomas. An immunohistologic analysis demonstrating the value of LeuM1 antigen. Am J Pathol 1986;123:212–9.

269. _____, Battifora H, Burke JS, Rappaport H. Leu-M1 antigen in human neoplasms. An immunohistologic study of 400 cases. Am J Surg Pathol 1986;10:227–36.

270. _____, Esteban JM, Bailey A, Battifora H, Weiss LM. Immunopathologic and molecular studies as an aid to the diagnosis of malignant mesothelioma. Hum Pathol 1992;23:107–16.

271. _____, Shin SS, Kezirian J, Weiss LM. Ber-EP4 antibody as a discriminant in the differential diagnosis of malignant mesothelioma vs. adenocarcinoma. Am J Surg Pathol 1991;15:779–84.

272. Sherman ME, Mark EJ. Effusion cytology in the diagnosis of malignant epithelioid and biphasic pleural mesothelioma. Arch Pathol Lab Med 1990;114:845–51.

273. Singer S, Boddington MM, Hudson EA. Immunocytochemical reaction of Ca1 and HMFG2 monoclonal antibodies with cells from serous effusions. J Clin Pathol 1985;38:180–4.

274. Situnayake RD, Middleton WG. Recurrent pneumothorax and malignant pleural mesothelioma. Respir Med 1991;85:255–6.

275. Sloane JP, Ormerod MG. Distribution of epithelial membrane antigen in normal and neoplastic tissues and its value in diagnostic tumor pathology. Cancer 1981;47:1786–95.

276. Smith MJ, Naylor B. A method for extracting ferruginous bodies from sputum and pulmonary tissue. Am J Clin Pathol 1972;58:250–4.

277. Smith WE, Miller L, Elsasser RE, Hubert DD. Tests for carcinogenicity of asbestos. Ann NY Acad Sci 1965;132:456–88.

278. Solomon A. Radiological features of diffuse mesothelioma. Environ Res 1970;3:330–8.

279. Soosay GN, Griffiths M, Papadaki L, Happerfield L, Bobrow L. The differential diagnosis of epithelial-type mesothelioma from adenocarcinoma and reactive mesothelial proliferation. J Pathol 1991;163:299–305.

280. Sridhar KS, Doria R, Raub WA Jr, Thurer RJ, Saldana M. New strategies are needed in diffuse malignant mesothelioma. Cancer 1992;70:2969–79.

281. Stanton MF, Wrench C. Mechanisms of mesothelioma induction with asbestos and fibrous glass. JNCI 1972;48:797–821.

282. Stanton W. Some etiological considerations of fibre carcinogenesis. In: Bogovski P, Gilson JG, Timbrell V, Wagner JC, eds. Biological effects of asbestos. Lyon: International Agency for Research on Cancer, 1973:289–94.

283. Steinetz C, Clarke R, Jacobs GH, Abdul-Karim FW, Petrelli M, Tomashefski JF Jr. Localized fibrous tumors of the pleura: correlation of histopathological, immunohistochemical and ultrastructural features. Path Res Pract 1990;186:344–57.

284. Stirling JW, Henderson DW, Spagnolo DV, Whitaker D. Unusual granular reactivity for carcinoembryonic antigen in malignant mesothelioma. Hum Pathol 1990;21:678–9.

285. Stock RJ, Fu YS, Carter JR. Malignant peritoneal mesothelioma following radiotherapy for seminoma of the testis. Cancer 1979;44:914–9.

286. Stout AP, Murray MR. Localized pleural mesothelioma. Arch Pathol 1942;34:951–64.

287. Strickler JG, Herndier BG, Rouse RV. Immunohistochemical staining in malignant mesotheliomas. Am J Clin Pathol 1987;88:610–4.

288. Sugarbaker DJ, Strauss GM, Lynch TJ, et al. Node status has prognostic significance in the multimodality therapy of diffuse, malignant mesothelioma. J Clin Oncol 1993;11:1172–8.

289. Sussman J, Rosai J. Lymph node metastasis as the initial manifestation of malignant mesothelioma: report of six cases. Am J Surg Pathol 1990;14:819–28.

290. Suzuki Y. Pathology of human malignant mesothelioma. Semin Oncol 1981;8:268–82.

291. _____, Kannerstein M. Ultrastructure of human malignant diffuse mesothelioma. Am J Pathol 1976;85:241–62.

292. _____, Kohyama N. Malignant mesothelioma induced by asbestos and zeolite in the mouse peritoneal cavity. Environ Res 1984;35:277–92.

293. Szpak CA, Johnston WW, Lottich SC, Kufe D, Thor A, Schlom J. Patterns of reactivity of four novel monoclonal antibodies (B72.3, DF3, B1.1 and B6.2) with cells in human malignant and benign effusions. Acta Cytol 1984;28:356–67.

294. _____, Johnston WW, Roggli V, et al. The diagnostic distinction between malignant mesothelioma of the pleura and adenocarcinoma of the lung as defined by a monoclonal antibody (B72.3). Am J Pathol 1986;122:252–60.

295. Takiyama Y, Tempero MA, Takasaki H, et al. Reactivity of CO17-1A and B72.3 in benign and malignant pancreatic diseases. Hum Pathol 1989;20:832–8.

296. Talerman A, Montero JR, Chilcote RR, Okagaki T. Diffuse malignant peritoneal mesothelioma in a 13-year-old girl. Report of a case and review of the literature. Am J Surg Pathol 1985;9:73–80.

297. Tao L. The cytopathology of mesothelioma. Acta Cytol 1979;23:209–13.

298. Taryle DA, Lakshminarayan S, Sahn SA. Pleural mesotheliomas—an analysis of 18 cases and review of the literature. Medicine 1976;55:153–62.

299. Terao K. Mesotheliomas induced by sterigmatocystin in Wistar rats. Gann 1978;69:237–47.

300. Thomas P, Battifora H. Keratins versus epithelial membrane antigen in tumor diagnosis: an immunohistochemical comparison of five monoclonal antibodies. Hum Pathol 1987;18:728–34.

301. Thor A, Gorstein F, Ohuchi N, Szpak CA, Johston WW, Schlom J. Tumor-associated glycoprotein (TAG-72) in ovarian carcinomas defined by monoclonal antibody B72.3. JNCI 1986;76:995–1006.

302. Tiainen M, Hopman A, Moesker O, et al. Interphase cytogenetics on paraffin sections of malignant pleural mesothelioma. A comparison to conventional karyotyping and flow cytometric studies. Cancer Genet Cytogenet 1992;62:171–9.

303. Timbrell V. Physical factors as etiological mechanisms. In: Bogovski P, Gilson JG, Timbrell V, Wagner JC, eds. Biological effects of asbestos. Lyon: IARC Sci Publ 1973:295–303.

304. Tron V, Wright JL, Churg A. Carcinoembryonic antigen and milk-fat globule protein staining of malignant mesothelioma and adenocarcinoma of the lung. Arch Pathol Lab Med 1987;111:291–3.

305. Tuomi T, Huuskonen MS, Tammilehto L, Vanhala E, Virtamo M. Occupational exposure to asbestos as evaluated from work histories and analysis of lung tissues from patients with mesothelioma. Br J Ind Med 1991;48:48–52.

306. Umsawasdi T, Dhingra HM, Charnsangavej C, Luna MA. A case report of malignant pleural mesothelioma with long-term disease control after chemotherapy. Cancer 1991;67:48–54.

307. Viallat JR, Raybaud F, Passarel M, Boutin C. Pleural migration of chrysotile fibres after intratracheal injection in rats. Arch Envir Health 1986;41:282–6.

308. Vianna NJ, Polan AK. Non-occupational exposure to asbestos and malignant mesothelioma in females. Lancet 1978;1:1061–3.

309. Vogelzang NJ. Malignant mesothelioma: diagnostic and management strategies for 1992. Semin Oncol 1992;19 (Suppl)11:64–71.

310. Wagner JC. Experimental production of mesothelial tumours of the pleura by implantation of dusts in laboratory animals. Nature 1962;196:180–1.

311. _____, Griffiths DM, Munday DE. Recent investigations in animals and humans. In: Wagner JC, ed. Accomplishments in oncology; the biological effects of chrysotile. Lyon: IARC Sci Publ, 1987:111–20.

312. _____, Sleggs CA, Marchand P. Diffuse pleural mesothelioma and asbestos exposure in the North Western Cape Province. Br J Ind Med 1960;17:260–71.

313. Walker AN, Mills SE. Surgical pathology of tunica vaginalis testis and embryologically related mesothelium. Pathol Ann 1988;23:125–52.

314. Walker C, Everitt J, Barrett JC. Possible cellular and molecular mechanisms for asbestos carcinogenicity. Am J Ind Med 1992;21:253–73.

315. Walts AE, Said JW, Banks-Schlegel SP. Keratin and carcinoembryonic antigen in exfoliated mesothelial and malignant cells: an immunoperoxidase study. Am J Clin Pathol 1983;80:671–6.

316. _____, Said JW, Shintaku PI, Sassoon AF, Banks-Schlegel SP. Keratins of different molecular weight in exfoliated mesothelial and adenocarcinoma cells—an aid to cell identification. Am J Clin Pathol 1984;81:442–6.

317. Wanebo HJ, Martini N, Melamed MR, Hilaris B, Beattie E. Pleural mesothelioma. Cancer 1976;38:2481–8.

318. Wang NS, Huang SN, Gold P. Absence of carcinoembryonic antigen-like material in mesothelioma: an immunohistochemical differentiation from other lung cancers. Cancer 1979;44:937–43.

319. Warhol MJ. Electron microscopy and the diagnosis of mesothelioma with routine biopsy, needle biopsy and fluid cytology. In: Antman K, Aisner J, eds. Asbestos-related malignancy. Orlando: Grune and Stratton, 1987:201–24.

320. Warhol MJ, Corson JM. An ultrastructural comparison of mesotheliomas with adenocarcinoms of the lung and breast. Hum Pathol 1985;16:50–55.

321. _____, Hickey WF, Corson JM. Malignant mesothelioma: ultrastructural distinction from adenocarcinoma. Am J Surg Pathol 1982;6:307–14.

322. Warnock ML, Stoloff A, Thor A. Differentiation of adenocarcinoma of the lung from mesothelioma. Periodic acid-Schiff, monoclonal antibodies B72.3, and Leu M1. Am J Pathol 1988;133:30–8.

323. Wassermann M, Wassermann D, Steinitz R, Katz L, Lemesch C. Mesothelioma in children. In: Wagner JC, ed. Biological effect of mineral fibres. Lyon: IARC Sci Publ 1980:253–7.

324. Waxler B, Eisenstein R, Battifora H. Electrophoresis of tissue glycosaminoglycans as an aid in the diagnosis of mesothelioma. Cancer 1979;44:221–7.

325. Weiss A. Pleurakrebs bein Lungenasbestose, in vivo morphologisch gesichert. Medizinische 1953;1:93–4.

326. Weiss SW, Tavassoli FA. Multicystic mesothelioma. An analysis of pathologic findings and biologic behavior in 37 cases. Am J Surg Pathol 1988;12:737–46.

327. Whitaker D, Henderson DW, Shilkin KB. The concept of mesothelioma in situ: implications for diagnosis and histogenesis. Sem Diag Pathol 1992;9:151–61.

328. _____, Manning LS, Robinson DW, Shilkin KB. The pathobiology of mesothelium. In: Henderson DW, Shilkin KB, Langlois SL, Whitaker D, eds. Malignant mesothelioma. New York: Hemisphere Publishing, 1992:25–56.

329. _____, Shilkin KB, Sterrett GF. Cytological appearances of malignant mesothelioma. In: Henderson DW, Shilkin KB, Langlois SL, Whitaker D, eds. Malignant mesothelioma. New York: Hemisphere Publishing, 1992:167–82.

330. _____, Sterrett GF, Shilkin K. Detection of tissue CEA-like substance as an aid in the differential diagnosis of malignant mesothelioma. Pathology 1982;14:255–8.

331. Whitwell F, Rawcliffe RM. Diffuse malignant pleural meso-thelioma and asbestos exposure. Thorax 1971;26:6–22.

332. Wick MR, Loy T, Mills SE, Legier JF, Manivel JC. Malignant epithelioid pleural mesothelioma versus peripheral pulmonary adenocarcinoma: a histochemical, ultrastructural, and immunohistologic study of 103 cases. Hum Pathol 1990;21:759–66.

333. _____, Mills SE, Swanson PE. Expression of myelomonocytic antigens in mesotheliomas and adenocarcinomas involving the serosal surfaces. Am J Clin Pathol 1990;94:18–26.

334. Wignall BK, Fox AJ. Mortality of female gas mask assemblers. Br J Ind Med 1982;39:34–8.

335. Wilson GE, Hasleton PS, Chatterjee AK. Desmoplastic malignant mesothelioma: a review of 17 cases. J Clin Pathol 1992;45:295–8.

336. Winslow DJ, Taylor HB. Malignant peritoneal mesotheliomas. A clinicopathological analysis of 12 fatal cases. Cancer 1960;13:127–36.

337. Wirth PR, Legier J, Wright GL Jr. Immunohistochemical evaluation of seven monoclonal antibodies for differentiation of pleural mesothelioma from lung adenocarcinoma. Cancer 1991;67:655–62.

338. World Health Organization. Man-made mineral fibres. In: WHO, ed. Environmental health criteria. Geneva: World Health Organization, 1988:16–19.

339. Wrba F, Fertl H, Amann G, Tell E, Krepler R. Epithelial markers in synovial sarcoma. An immunohistochemical study on paraffin embedded tissues. Virchows Arch [A] 1989;415:253–8.

340. Wu Y, Parker LM, Binder NE, et al. The mesothelial keratins: a new family of cytoskeletal proteins identified in cultured mesothelial cells and nonkeratinizing epithelia. Cell 1982;31:693–703.

341. Yap BS, Benjamin RS, Burgess MA, Bodey GP. The value of adriamycin in the treatment of diffuse malignant pleural mesothelioma. Cancer 1978;42:1692–6.

342. Yesner R, Hurwitz A. Localized pleural mesothelioma of epithelial type. J Thorac Surg 1953;26:325–9.

343. Yokoi T, Mark EJ. Atypical mesothelial hyperplasia associated with bronchogenic carcinoma. Hum Pathol 1991;22:695–9.

344. Young RH, Scully RE. Testicular and paratesticular tumors and tumor-like lesions of ovarian common epithelial and mullerian types. A report of four cases and review of the literature. Am J Clin Pathol 1986;86:146–52.

345. Yousem SA, Hochholzer L. Malignant mesotheliomas with osseous and cartilaginous differentiation. Arch Pathol Lab Med 1987;111:62–6.

346. _____, Hochholzer L. Unusual thoracic manifestations of epithelioid hemangioendothelioma. Arch Pathol Lab Med 1987;111:459–63.

347. Zielhuis RL, Versteeg JP, Planteydt HT. Pleura mesothelioma and exposure to asbestos. Int Arch Occup Environ Health 1975;36:1–18.

✧ ✧ ✧

5

OTHER TUMORS AND LESIONS OF MESOTHELIAL ORIGIN

SEROUS NEOPLASIA OF THE PERITONEUM

Diffuse malignant mesothelioma (DMM) has a remarkable range of histologic and cytologic characteristics. The spectrum assumes an added dimension when it is recalled that serous neoplasms, the most common and diverse group of epithelial tumors in the ovary, are also of mesothelial origin. Spanning the middle ground between DMM and ovarian serous tumor is a group of primary serous papillary tumors of the peritoneum that occur mainly in women. These tumors may resemble, histologically, DMM of tubulopapillary type or serous papillary tumors of the ovary, or they may be intermediate between the two (14). The resemblance to serous ovarian tumors appears to reflect the existence of a secondary Müllerian system (24,25), as does the proclivity for well-differentiated papillary mesothelioma to develop in the female peritoneum. This secondary system embraces mesothelium covering ovary and peritoneum that has the potential to produce metaplastic or neoplastic epithelial elements resembling those found in various parts of the primary Müllerian system.

The variable characteristics and associations of primary peritoneal serous papillary tumors, and the extent to which their behavior is linked to their differentiation, have important prognostic, therapeutic, and epidemiologic implications. The pathology of these serous tumors, as well as that of the miscellaneous mesothelial entities known as well-differentiated papillary mesothelioma, benign multicystic mesothelioma, (multilocular peritoneal inclusion cyst), adenomatoid tumor, and peritoneal transitional cell lesions are outlined in this section. Reference is also made to a neoplasm known as "intra-abdominal desmoplastic small round-cell tumor" that is possibly of mesothelial origin (16). There is no evidence that asbestos is causally related to any of these forms of serosal neoplasm or mesothelial tumor although the authors are not aware of any epidemiologic study concerning this.

PRIMARY SEROUS PAPILLARY CARCINOMA OF THE PERITONEUM

Primary serous papillary carcinoma of peritoneum (PSCP) closely resembles ovarian serous papillary carcinoma histologically, and may occur in women whose ovaries are free of tumor or have only small granules of tumor on the ovarian surface (14,23). It may also occur in ovarian cancer–prone families after prophylactic oophorectomy (48). The most common presenting manifestations are abdominal pain and distension (41). The manner in which the peritoneum is involved and the behavior of PSCP are often similar to DMM and the extraovarian component of stage III ovarian serous carcinoma, although occasionally the tumor forms dominant localized masses (23,49). Microscopically, a papillary or tubulopapillary pattern is usually conspicuous (fig. 5-1) and psammoma bodies are sometimes numerous (fig. 5-2). The cells lining the papillary and tubular elements in the better-differentiated tumors may show the budding or tufting that occurs in borderline malignant or well-differentiated malignant ovarian serous tumors (fig. 5-3). The tumor cells tend to be smaller and more crowded, and to have more hematoxyphilic nuclei than those of DMM. Cytoplasmic granules stain with periodic acid–Schiff after diastase digestion in many instances (14). PSCP is differentiated from DMM by the use of panels of immunohistochemical stains (see Table 4-10). Some investigators have found that the prognosis for PSCP is worse than for ovarian serous cancers with a comparable degree of peritoneal spread (21,37); others have found no significant difference (8,15,41). The median survival time is from 11 to 24 months (41).

Some PSCPs have the histopathologic features of ovarian serous papillary tumors of "borderline malignancy" (low malignant potential) (3,4,32). With few exceptions, these low malignant potential tumors have an excellent prognosis, even when untreated (3,4). The tumor appears grossly as multiple adhesions or granular lesions of the peritoneum, and the ovarian surfaces are often involved (2). In addition to tumor, endosalpingiosis is commonly present and benign ovarian serous

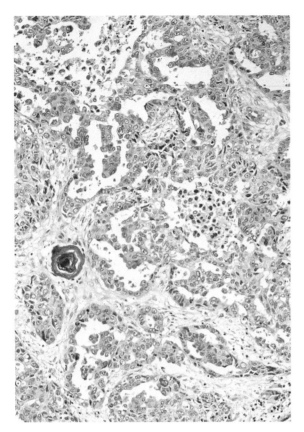

Figure 5-1
PRIMARY SEROUS PAPILLARY TUMOR
OF THE PERITONEUM
Example of a case showing tubular and papillary pattern.

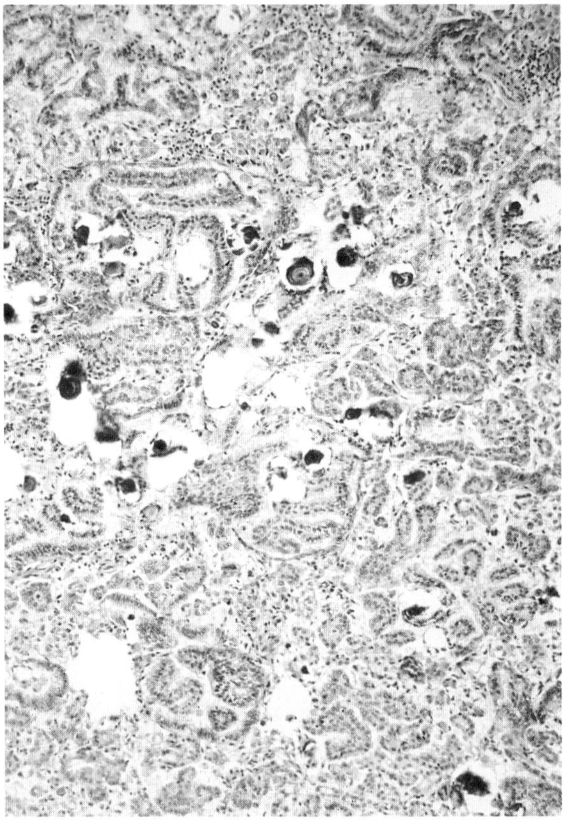

Figure 5-2
PRIMARY SEROUS PAPILLARY TUMOR
OF THE PERITONEUM
Abundant psammoma bodies are present.

tumor masses (serous cystadenomas) are found (fig. 5-4)(3). *Serous psammocarcinoma of peritoneum* is a rare variant of PSCP characterized by massive psammoma body formation (fig. 5-5) and low-grade cytologic features (18,34). These tumors behave in an indolent fashion, even when lymphatic invasion is extensive (fig. 5-6)(34). Serous tumors of low malignant potential occasionally arise in the broad ligament (7).

BENIGN MULTICYSTIC MESOTHELIOMA

This rare lesion mainly arises from the pelvic peritoneum and may involve the surfaces of the uterus, ovary, bladder, rectum, or cul de sac. It often forms a large multicystic mass (fig. 5-7) but extension into the abdominal cavity in a discontinuous manner frequently occurs and occasionally the retroperitoneum is involved. Cystic lesions with these characteristics have been

described by various synonyms of which *multilocular peritoneal inclusion cyst* (42) is probably the most widely used at the present time. To date, around 130 cases of benign multicystic mesothelioma of peritoneum (BMMP) have been documented in the literature (42,50). While occurring predominantly in younger women (mean age, 37 years), the lesion has been described in an infant and in patients in their 60s (50). Around 17 percent of these tumors occur in men. A similar lesion has been described in the pleural cavity (1).

Patients usually present with chronic pelvic or abdominal pain and on examination often have a palpable abdominal mass which may be tender. However, lesions of this type are sometimes found incidentally at laparotomy in the form of single or multiple unilocular thin-walled cysts, which may be attached to serosa or free in the abdominal cavity (fig. 5-8). Of 37 reported cases, the lesions

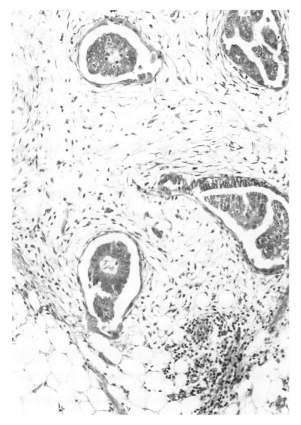

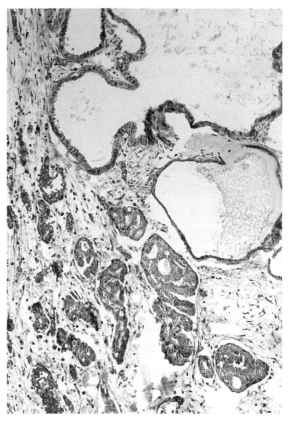

Figure 5-3
PRIMARY SEROUS PAPILLARY TUMOR
OF THE PERITONEUM
This pattern resembles that commonly exhibited by perito-
neal involvement by borderline serous tumor of ovarian origin.

Figure 5-4
PRIMARY SEROUS PAPILLARY TUMOR
OF THE PERITONEUM
This tumor is associated with endosalpingiosis. The
larger cystic spaces are lined by ciliated columnar epithe-
lium resembling tubal epithelium.

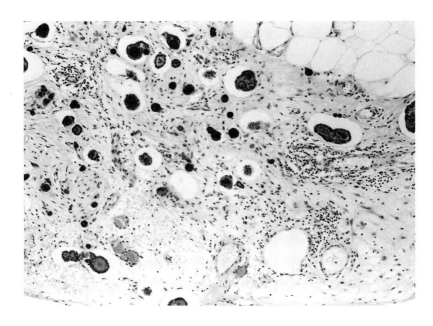

Figure 5-5
PRIMARY SEROUS PAPILLARY
TUMOR OF THE PERITONEUM
Massive psammoma body formation.

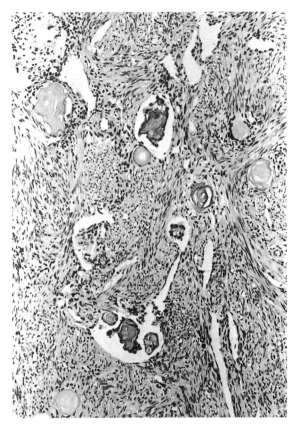

Figure 5-6
PRIMARY SEROUS PAPILLARY TUMOR
OF THE PERITONEUM
Extensive invasion of myometrial lymphatics by neoplastic cells.

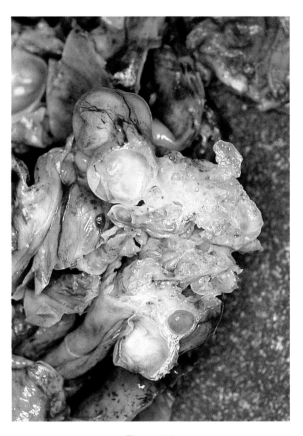

Figure 5-7
BENIGN MULTICYSTIC MESOTHELIOMA
Typical gross appearance. (Courtesy of Dr. R. H. Young, Boston, MA.)

were solitary in 6, localized and multifocal in 15, and diffuse in 16 (50). Rarely, BMMP may be found within hernia sacs (28) and we have occasionally seen it at the distal part of the round ligament. In rare cases it has been reported to involve the spleen, liver, or pancreas (50).

Typically, the lesions of BMMP consist of multiple, translucent, membranous cysts, often arranged in grape-like clusters and separated by varying amounts of fibrous tissue; they frequently group together to form a discontinuous studding of the surface of the peritoneum. The cysts range in diameter from a few millimeters to 20 cm. The intracystic fluid may be clear or blood-tinged, and occasionally mucinous or gelatinous.

Characteristically, the cysts are lined by one to several layers of flat to cuboidal cells (fig. 5-9) which possess the ultrastructural features of mesothelial cells. Hobnail-shaped cells are occa-

sionally seen (fig. 5-10). Foci of epithelial hyperplasia may be noted; rarely, squamous metaplasia is present (42). The cysts are separated by fibrous septa which may contain areas of acute and chronic inflammation, sometimes in association with necrosis, fibrin deposition, and granulation tissue (42). Areas of mural mesothelial proliferation are frequently seen in which the mesothelial cells form tubules, nests, or cords, and in some cases simulate an adenomatoid tumor (fig. 5-11) (35). As some cytologic atypia is also often present, these tumors occasionally have been misdiagnosed as serous carcinoma or malignant mesothelioma (35).

The most important entity in the differential diagnosis is cystic malignant mesothelioma. Occasional DMMs have grossly visible cystic foci and extensive microcystic changes. However, the gross characteristics of the lesion and the degree

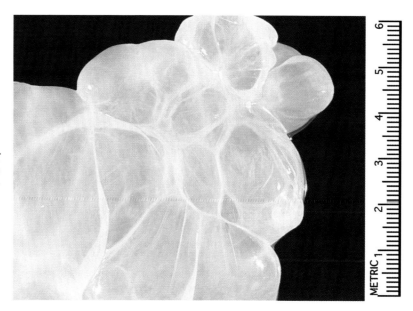

Figure 5-8
BENIGN MULTICYSTIC
MESOTHELIOMA
Grape-like translucent clusters of
vesicles in another example of cystic
mesothelioma. (Courtesy of Dr. R. H.
Young, Boston, MA.)

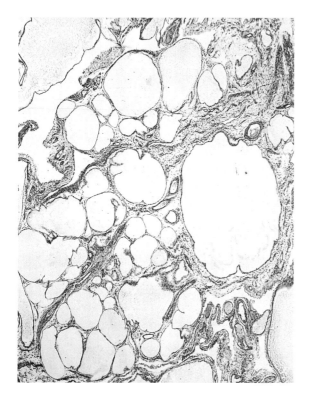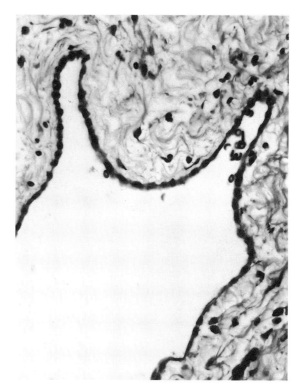

Figure 5-9
BENIGN MULTICYSTIC MESOTHELIOMA
Left: Numerous mesothelial-lined cysts embedded in a delicate fibrous stroma.
Right: Detail of one of the cysts. (Figs. 3 and 4b from Weiss SW, Tavassoli FA. Multicystic mesothelioma. An analysis of pathologic findings and biologic behavior in 37 cases. Am J Surg Pathol 1988;12:737–46.)

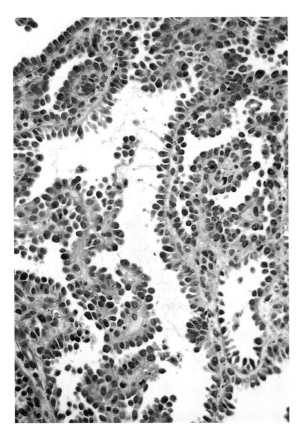

Figure 5-10
BENIGN MULTICYSTIC MESOTHELIOMA
Presence of hobnail-shaped cells in area of epithelial meso-thelioma within a multicystic mesothelioma. (Fig. 11B from Weiss SW, Tavassoli FA. Multicystic mesothelioma. An analysis of pathologic findings and biologic behavior in 37 cases. Am J Surg Pathol 1988;12:737–46.)

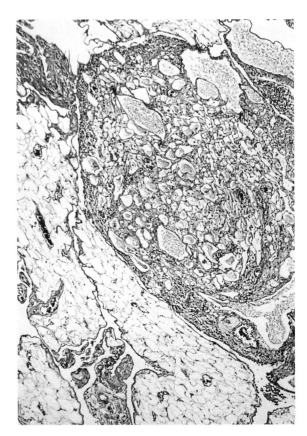

Figure 5-11
BENIGN MULTICYSTIC MESOTHELIOMA
Area simulating an adenomatoid tumor.

of cellular proliferation and atypia should permit ready differentiation of DMM and BMMP in most cases. Cystic lymphangioma may resemble BMMP grossly but usually is easily distinguished from it microscopically by the presence of smooth muscle and aggregates of lymphocytes in the lymphangi-oma wall. Immunohistochemically, the cyst lining cells of lymphangioma are sometimes immunoreac-tive for factor VIII–related antigen, but unlike the lining cells of BMMP they do not express keratin. Ultrastructurally, microvillous processes, desmo-somes, and tonofilaments, so typical of mesothelial lesions, are not observed in lymphangioma. Con-fusion with angiosarcoma of serous membranes (fig. 5-12) is also possible (33). Adenomatoid tu-mors may occasionally be cystic (22,40) and poten-tially could be confused with BMMP.

BMMP is usually clinically benign. However, approximately half recur at intervals ranging between 1 and 27 years (42). A few patients die of the disease (50). The progressive growth of the lesion and frequent recurrence suggests that it is a neoplasm, but the common history of previ-ous abdominal surgery, endometriosis, or pelvic inflammatory disease raises the possibility of a reactive origin (42,50).

ADENOMATOID TUMOR

This term was introduced in 1945 to describe a distinctive benign tumor that is nearly always found in relation to the genital tract (19). Ranging from a few millimeters to several centimeters in size, it is usually discrete, oval, or flattened, and grey, tan, or yellow. In males, most are located in the region of the epididymis, but a few occur in the spermatic cord or on the surface of the testis re-mote from the epididymis. In females, the majority

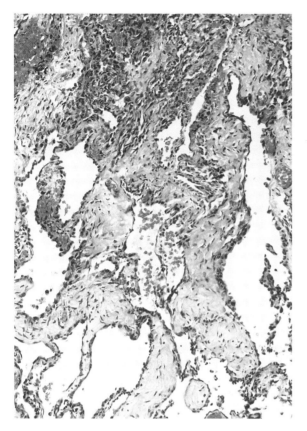

Figure 5-12
ANGIOSARCOMA OF THE PERITONEUM

Cavernous vascular spaces lined by atypical endothelial cells which are flattened in many places. Distinction from cystic mesothelioma may be greatly facilitated by immunohistochemical study.

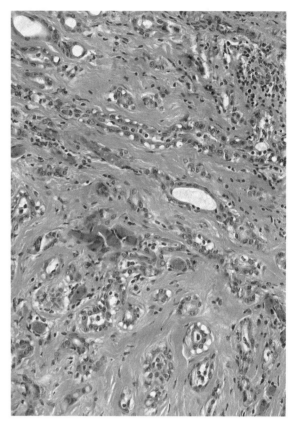

Figure 5-13
ADENOMATOID TUMOR

There is a predominant tubular pattern. Note the marked vacuolation of many of the tumor cells.

lie in relation to the fallopian tube, broad ligament, or serosal surface of uterus near the cornua but ovarian hilus and ovary have also been involved (52). Occasional tumors of similar histologic type have been described in the omentum (6,44). It has also been suggested that some tumors reported as lymphangiomas of adrenal gland are adenomatoid tumors.

Adenomatoid tumors contain plump acidophilic cells arranged in cords and tubules. Adenoid, angiomatoid, solid, and cystic histologic types have been recognized (40). Vacuolation of the cells, sometimes in a signet ring formation, is frequently seen and it has been suggested that coalescence of these vacuoles brings about the formation of the tubular spaces that are frequently found in the tumor (fig. 5-13). The cells lining these spaces are usually flattened or cuboi-

dal. The stroma is basically fibrous, but smooth muscle cells are sometimes present and may occasionally be very prominent. This smooth muscle proliferation is thought to be a non-neoplastic hyperplasia (40). A few adenomatoid tumors have infiltrated adjacent tissues (36) or have been multicentric, but malignant behavior is rare (46). Occasional tumors have been of giant proportions (10) and an example of giant cystic adenomatoid tumor has been described (5).

Although it has been suggested that these tumors are of lymphatic origin or derived from vestigial mesonephric or Müllerian elements, most ultrastructural studies have shown the tumor cells to have mesothelial characteristics (27,43,47). Other evidence supporting a mesothelial origin comes from the observation of similar areas in DMM (13) and immunohistochemical studies showing that the tumor cells express

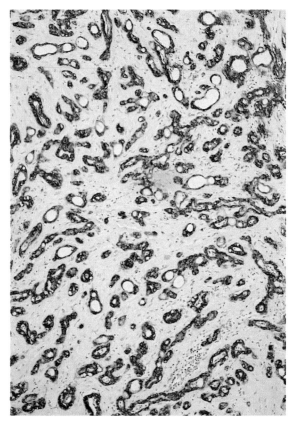

Figure 5-14
ADENOMATOID TUMOR
This was stained with a cocktail of monoclonal antibodies to low molecular weight cytokeratins. Strong immunoreactivity of virtually every cell is noted. This suffices to rule out an endothelial origin.

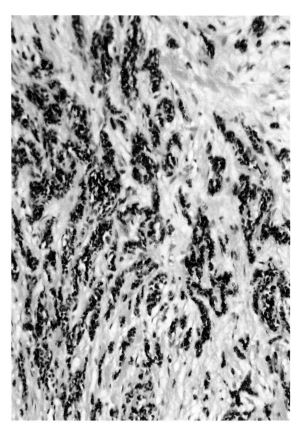

Figure 5-15
INTRA-ABDOMINAL DESMOPLASTIC
ROUND CELL TUMOR
This example was from a large retroperitoneal mass in a 27-year-old man.

cytokeratin (fig. 5-14) (47). Earlier reports stating that some tumors express factor VIII–related antigen, and were thus of endothelial origin, have not been confirmed and probably represent false positive results due to the presence of cross-reacting natural antibodies in the rabbit antisera used for most of these studies. These adenomatoid tumors are best described as *adenomatoid mesotheliomas* (9).

INTRA-ABDOMINAL DESMOPLASTIC ROUND CELL TUMOR

This distinctive type of peritoneal tumor has clinical, topographic, morphologic, and immuno-histochemical features that set it apart from all of the well-recognized members of the family of small round cell tumors of infancy and childhood (16). The possibility that this tumor might be of

mesothelial origin has been suggested (16). It is also known as *desmoplastic small cell tumor with divergent differentiation* (17,20). This unusual tumor usually occurs in males between 8 and 30 years of age and typically presents at laparotomy as a large intra-abdominal mass with smaller peritoneal "implants" (16). Microscopically, the most distinctive finding on low-power examination is sharply outlined basophilic clusters of tumor cells embedded in a desmoplastic fibrous stroma (fig. 5-15) (16,20). The tumor cell clusters may appear epithelial, but when the tumor cells are smaller, the appearance, excepting the prominent stroma, may be highly reminiscent of the small cell tumors of infancy. Focal rhabdoid features and clear cell change may be seen. Immunohistochemically, reactivity for epithelial (keratin, epithelial membrane antigen [EMA]), neural (neuron-specific enolase

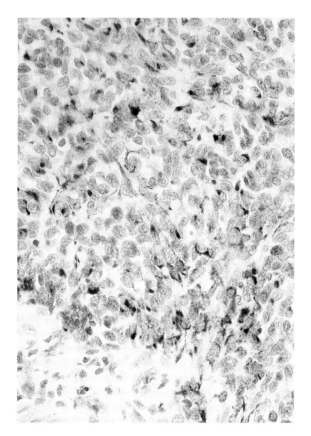

Figure 5-16
INTRA-ABDOMINAL DESMOPLASTIC
ROUND CELL TUMOR
Staining with a monoclonal antibody to desmin shows a punctate paranuclear mass of desmin filaments in many of the tumor cells.

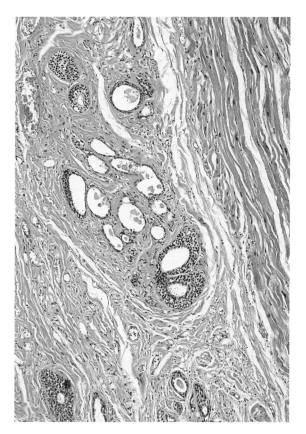

Figure 5-17
"MESOTHELIOMA" OF THE
ATRIOVENTRICULAR NODE
Typical example from a man who died unexpectedly. There were intraluminal deposits of amorphous material that was mucicarminophilic. The cells were positive for Leu-M1 (CD15) and CEA, and there was a strong cytoplasmic pattern for HMFG-2 and EMA.

[NSE]), and muscle (desmin) markers are commonly seen; the latter are often in a dot-like paranuclear pattern (fig. 5-16). An interesting and diagnostically useful immunophenotypic feature is the absence of detectable smooth muscle actin, despite the presence of readily demonstrable desmin, unlike other muscle-derived tumors (16). Ultrastructurally, a notable feature is the presence of intermediate cytoplasmic filaments, often packed in perinuclear bundles or whorls. Dense core granules are seen in a few cases (16). In rare cases, small intracellular lumina containing short microvilli are seen (39). The tumors are usually highly aggressive. The possibility that they are of mesothelial origin has been suggested because of the diffuse peritoneal pattern of spread, the presence of epithelial differentiation in the tumor cells, and the fact that fetal mesothelium coexpresses keratin and desmin. The

observation that NSE is expressed by some round cell tumors is also consistent with DMM, as mesotheliomas, including a small cell variant, frequently express NSE (29,30). It has been suggested that these tumors may be blastomas arising from intraembryonic mesoderm or coelom and the nosologic entity of "mesothelioblastoma" has been proposed (51).

"MESOTHELIOMA" OF THE ATRIOVENTRICULAR NODE

Often identified as the smallest tumor that causes sudden death, the "mesothelioma" of the atrioventricular node is now believed to be neither a tumor nor a mesothelioma. The typical lesion measures a few millimeters and consists of small cysts and nests lined by cuboidal or columnar cells (fig. 5-17). Some cysts have attenuated epithelium and thus resemble adenomatoid tumor (31). Mucin may be present in the lumina. The boundary with the adjacent myocardium is not well defined and blending of the two types of tissue is not unusual. Earlier ultrastructural studies led to the false conclusion that these lesions were of mesothelial origin (12,31). Although microvilli can be seen on the surface of the epithelial nests, they are sparse and short. Several histochemical and immunohistochemical studies have shown production of hyaluronidase-resistant neutral mucin and carcinoembryonic antigen (CEA) (11,26,38,45).

Currently, this lesion is considered to represent congenital heterotopia of endodermal tissues in the atrioventricular node.

REFERENCES

1. Ball NJ, Urbanski SJ, Green FH, Kieser T. Pleural multicystic mesothelial proliferation: the so-called multicystic mesothelioma. Am J Surg Pathol 1990;14:375–88.
2. Bell DA, Scully RE. Benign and borderline serous lesions of the peritoneum in women. Pathol Ann 1989;24:1–21.
3. _____, Scully RE. Serous borderline tumors of the peritoneum. Am J Surg Pathol 1990;14:230–9.
4. Biscotti CV, Hart WR. Peritoneal serous micropapillomatosis of low malignant (potential serous borderline tumors of the peritoneum). A clinical pathologic study of 17 cases. Am J Pathol 1992;16:467–75.
5. Bisset DL, Morris JA, Fox H. Giant cystic adenomatoid tumour (mesothelioma) of the uterus. Histopathology 1988;12:555–8.
6. Craig JR, Hart WR. Extragenital adenomatoid tumor: evidence for the mesothelial theory of origin. Cancer 1979;43:1678–81.
7. d'Ablaing G III, Klatt EC, DiRocco G, Hibbard LT. Broad ligament serous tumor of low malignant potential. Int J Gynecol Pathol 1983;2:93–9.
8. Dalrymple JC, Bannatyne P, Russell P, et al. Extraovarian peritoneal serous papillary carcinoma. A clinicopathological study of 31 cases. Cancer 1989;64:110–5.
9. Davie CL, Tang CK. Are all adenomatoid tumors adeomatoid mesotheliomas? Hum Pathol 1981;12:360–9.
10. De Rosa G, Boscaino A, Terracciano LM, Giordano G. Giant adenomatoid tumors of the uterus. Int J Gynecol Pathol 1992;11:156–60.
11. Duray PH, Mark EJ, Barwick KW, Madri JA, Strom RL. Congenital polycystic tumor of the atrioventricular node. Autopsy study with immunohistochemical findings suggesting endodermal derivation. Arch Pathol Lab Med 1985;109:30–4.
12. Fenoglio JJ Jr, Jacobs DW, McAllister HA. Ultrastructure of the mesothelioma of the atrioventricular node. Cancer 1977;40:721–7.
13. Ferenczy A, Fenoglio J, Richart RM. Observations on benign mesothelioma of the genital tract (adenomatoid tumor). A comparative ultrastructural study. Cancer 1972;30:244–60.
14. Foyle A, Al-Jabi M, McCaughey WT. Papillary peritoneal tumors in women. Am J Surg Pathol 1981;5:241–9.
15. Fromm GL, Gershenson DM, Silva EG. Papillary serous carcinoma of the peritoneum. Obstet Gynecol 1990;75:89–95.
16. Gerald WL, Miller HK, Battifora H, Miettinen M, Silva EG, Rosai J. Intra-abdominal desmoplastic small round cell tumor. Report of 19 cases of a distinctive type of high-grade polyphenotypic malignancy affecting young individuals. Am J Surg Pathol 1991;15:499–513.
17. _____, Rosai J. Desmoplastic small-cell tumor of divergent differentiation. Pediat Pathol 1989;9:177–83.
18. Gilks CB, Bell DA, Scully RE. Serous psammocarcinoma of the ovary and peritoneum. Int J Gynecol Pathol 1990;9:110–21.
19. Golden A, Ash J. Adenomatoid tumors of genital tract. Am J Pathol 1945;21:63–80.
20. Gonzalez-Crussi F, Crawford SE, Sun CC. Intra-abdominal desmoplastic small-cell tumor of divergent differentiation. Observations on three cases of childhood. Am J Surg Pathol 1990;14:633–42.
21. Gooneratne S, Sassone M, Blaustein A, Talerman M. Serous surface papillary carcinoma of the ovary: a clinicopathologic study of 16 cases. Int J Gynecol Pathol 1982;1:258–69.
22. Iwasaki I, Yu TJ, Tamuru J, Asanuma K. A cystic adenomatoid tumor of the uterus simulating lymphangioma grossly. Acta Pathol Jpn 1985;35:989–93.
23. Kannerstein M, Churg J, McCaughey WT, Hill D. Papillary tumors of the peritoneum in women: mesothelioma or papillary carcinoma. Am J Obstet Gynecol 1977;127:306–14.
24. Lauchlan SC. Conceptual unity of the Müllerian tumor group. A histologic study. Cancer 1968;22:601
25. _____. The secondary Müllerian system. Obstet Gynecol Survey 1972;27:133–46.
26. Linder J, Shelburne JD, Sorge JP, Whalen RE, Hackel DB. Congenital endodermal heterotopia of the atrioventricular node: evidence for the endodermal origin of so-called mesotheliomas of atrioventricular node. Hum Pathol 1994;15:1093–8.
27. Mackay B, Bennington JL, Skoglund RW. The adenomatoid tumor: fine structural evidence for a mesothelial origin. Cancer 1971;27:109–15.
28. Marshall RM, Gould VE, King ME, Jensik S, Chejfec G. Multicystic abdominal peritoneal tumor presenting as an enlarging incisional hernia. Ultrastruct Pathol 1985;8:249–56.
29. Mayall FG, Gibbs AR. The histology and immunohistochemistry of small cell mesothelioma. Histopathology 1992;20:47–51.

30. _____, Jasani B, Gibbs AR. Immunohistochemical positivity for neuron-specific enolase and Leu-7 in malignant mesotheliomas. J Pathol 1991;165:325–28.

31. McAllister HA Jr, Fenoglio JJ Jr. Tumors of the cardiovascular system. Atlas of Tumor Pathology, 2nd Series, Fascicle 15. Washington DC: Armed Forces Institute of Pathology, 1978:52–8.

32. McCaughey WT. Papillary peritoneal neoplasms in females. Pathol Ann 1985;20:385–404.

33. _____, Dardick I, Barr JR. Angiosarcoma of serous membrane. Arch Pathol Lab Med 1983;107:304–7.

34. _____, Schryer MJ, Lin XS, Al-Jabi M. Extraovarian pelvic serous tumor with marked calcification. Arch Pathol Lab Med 1986;110:78–80.

35. McFadden DE, Clement PB. Peritoneal inclusion cysts with mural mesothelial proliferation. A clinical pathological analysis of six cases. Am J Surg Pathol 1986;10:844–54.

36. Miller F, Lieberman MK. Local invasion in adenomatoid tumors. Cancer 1968;21:933–9.

37. Mills SE, Andersen WA, Fechner RE, Austin MB. Serous surface papillary carcinoma. A clinicopathologic study of 10 cases and comparison to stage III–IV ovarian serous carcinoma. Am J Surg Pathol 1988;12:827–34.

38. Monma N, Satodate R, Tashiro A, Segawa I. Origin of so-called mesothelioma of the atrioventricular node. An immunohistochemical study. Arch Pathol Lab Med 1991;115:1026–9.

39. Ordóñez NG, Zirkin R, Bloom RE. Malignant small-cell epithelial tumor of the peritoneum coexpressing mesenchymal-type intermediate filaments. Am J Surg Pathol 1989;13:413–21.

40. Quigley JC, Hart WR. Adenomatoid tumors of the uterus. Am J Clin Pathol 1981;76:627–35.

41. Ransom DT, Patel SR, Keeney GL, Malkasion GD, Edmonson JH. Papillary serous carcinoma of the peritoneum. A review of 33 cases treated with platin-based chemotherapy. Cancer 1990;66:1091–4.

42. Ross MJ, Welch WR, Scully RE. Multilocular peritoneal inclusion cysts (so-called cystic mesothelioma). Cancer 1989;64:1336–46.

43. Salazar H, Kanbour A, Burgess F. Ultrastructure and observations on the histogenesis of mesotheliomas' adenomatoid tumors, of the female genital tract. Cancer 1972;29:141–52.

44. Soini Y, Turpeenniemi-Hujanen T, Kamel D, et al. p53 immunohistochemistry in transitional cell carcinoma and dysplasia of the urinary bladder correlates with disease progression. Br J Cancer 1993;68:1029–35.

45. Sopher IM, Spitz WU. Endodermal inclusions of the heart: so-called mesothelioma of the atrioventricular node. Arch Pathol 1971;92:180–6.

46. Söderström J, Liederberg CF. Malignant adenomatoid tumor of the epididymis. Acta Path Microbiol Immunol Scand 1966;67:165–8.

47. Stephenson TJ, Mills PM. Adenomatoid tumours: an immunohistochemical and ultrastructural appraisal of their histogenesis. J Pathol 1986;148:327–35.

48. Tobacman JK, Greene MH, Tucker MA, Costa J, Kase R, Fraumeni JF Jr. Intra-abdominal carcinomatosis after prophylactic oophorectomy in ovarian-cancer-prone families. Lancet 1982;795–7.

49. Ulbright TM, Morley DJ, Roth LM, Berkow RL. Papillary serous carcinoma of the retroperitoneum. Am J Clin Pathol 1983;79:633–7.

50. Weiss SW, Tavassoli FA. Multicystic mesothelioma. An analysis of pathologic findings and biologic behavior in 37 cases. Am J Surg Pathol 1988;12:737–46.

51. Yeoh G, Russell P, Wills EJ, Fleming S. Intra-abdominal desmoplastic small round cell tumor. Pathology 1993;25:197–202.

52. Young RH, Silva EG, Scully RE. Ovarian and juxtaovarian adenomatoid tumors: a report of six cases. Int J Gynecol Pathol 1991;10:364–71.

❖ ❖ ❖

6

TUMORS OF SUBMESOTHELIAL ORIGIN

These tumors are not regarded as being of mesothelial origin, but they may present as pleural-based neoplasms and are part of the mesothelioma differential diagnosis. Although the majority present as localized pleural or subpleural tumors, a few, particularly those of vascular origin (18), secondarily involve the pleural surfaces and closely resemble mesothelioma clinically and radiologically. By far the most important tumor in this group is a distinctive form of localized fibrous neoplasm (often called localized mesothelioma) that seems to have a more intimate relationship with the serous membranes than other tumors in this group. Benign and malignant mesenchymal tumors exhibiting neural, vascular, fibrous, adipose, or muscular differentiation may secondarily, although infrequently, involve the pleura and need to be distinguished from sarcomatoid mesothelioma. Also, focal heterologous mesenchymal metaplasia may be occasionally observed in otherwise bona fide mesotheliomas (2).

LOCALIZED FIBROUS TUMOR

Histogenesis. Localized fibrous tumors are also known as *localized (solitary) mesothelioma, pleural fibroma, submesothelial fibroma,* and *localized fibrous mesothelioma.* The gross and histologic attributes of these localized tumors are very different from those of sarcomatoid diffuse malignant mesothelioma (DMM), and this, together with evidence from ultrastructural and immunohistochemical studies, has led most researchers to conclude that localized fibrous tumor is not of mesothelial origin but arises in submesothelial connective tissue. A constant feature is the lack of cytokeratins in contrast with their consistent expression by sarcomatous mesothelioma (1,4,5,7,23). Thus, the pathway of differentiation of the spindle cells in localized fibrous tumor of the pleura is more akin to that of fibroblasts than to that of the submesothelial cells that play a role in the regeneration of the mesothelial surface. Occasional tumors of this type occur in sites (nasal and paranasal sinuses, mediastinum, retroperitoneum, lung parenchyma) that are either remote from or not in contact with serous membranes (14,28,30,31).

Etiology. There is no evidence of an epidemiologically significant association of localized fibrous tumor of the pleura with asbestos exposure or any other carcinogen, although we have seen occasional cases in persons exposed to asbestos.

Incidence. Localized fibrous tumor of the pleura is rare: only 2.8 cases per 100,000 registrations at the Mayo Clinic were recorded (20). Some observers find them to be more common than diffuse mesotheliomas (25); others find them less common (21). These discrepancies probably reflect geographic variations in the frequency of diffuse mesothelioma due to occupational or environmental influences.

Clinical Features. Localized fibrous tumor of the pleura may appear at any stage of life, including childhood (15). Although the proportions have varied in different studies, there is no evidence for a significant sex bias or predilection for either pleural cavity. About 50 percent of the cases are asymptomatic and the tumors are incidental discoveries on routine chest roentgenograms (3). Chest pain, cough, dyspnea, pulmonary osteoarthropathy, digital clubbing, and fever are the most common manifestations (10, 20). Larger tumors may give rise to ipsilateral pleural effusion or hypoglycemia (6). A few have been associated with galactorrhea (3). Hypoglycemia has also been described in mediastinal solitary fibrous tumors (28).

Chest X rays usually reveal a circumscribed and homogeneous lesion mainly located at the lung periphery or related to a fissure (20). Some tumors are pedunculated and a change in position associated with body movement may be demonstrated radiologically.

Gross Pathologic Findings. Two thirds of the tumors are attached to the visceral pleura, often by a pedicle (10); the remainder arise from the parietal, diaphragmatic, or mediastinal pleura. The tumors range from 1 to 36 cm in maximum diameter, with an average diameter of 6 cm (3). Occasional examples have weighed more that 3 kg (6,17). Approximately 80 percent

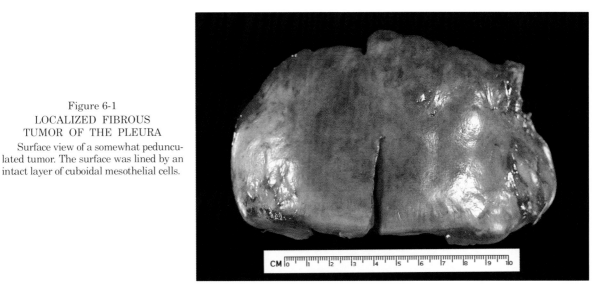

Figure 6-1
LOCALIZED FIBROUS
TUMOR OF THE PLEURA
Surface view of a somewhat pedunculated tumor. The surface was lined by an intact layer of cuboidal mesothelial cells.

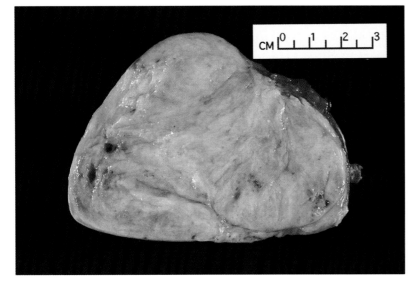

Figure 6-2
LOCALIZED FIBROUS
TUMOR OF THE PLEURA
Cut section of same tumor shown in figure 6-1. Note the focal areas of hemorrhage and the whorled pattern.

arise from visceral pleura and the remainder from the parietal pleura (3); rare cases have originated in the pericardium or peritoneum (9, 24,29). Frequently the tumor presents as a pedunculated mass lying entirely within the pleural cavity. When large, the tumors adhere to the pleural surfaces and their point of origin becomes obscured. A minority of localized fibrous tumors of the pleura project substantially within the lung substance and pleural cavity and occasional cases are entirely intrapulmonary (6,11, 20,30). The tumors are generally round, with the free surface often bosselated with a prominent superficial vasculature (fig. 6-1). Their interface with the lung parenchyma is sharply defined. The cut sections are commonly gray-white and may have a whorled pattern. Minute foci of hemorrhage or softening may be present (fig. 6-2).

Microscopic Findings. Fibrous areas of low to moderate cellularity are seen in most localized fibrous tumors of the pleura. In these areas, loosely arranged spindle-shaped or oval cells are scattered haphazardly among strands of collagen (fig. 6-3). At other times, however, there is a more distinctive distribution of the fibrous component characterized by abundant wire-like bands of hyalinized collagen that form complex anastomosing patterns (fig. 6-4). The histologic

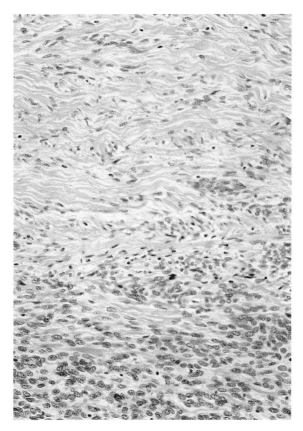

Figure 6-3
LOCALIZED FIBROUS TUMOR OF THE PLEURA
Cellular and highly collagenized areas.

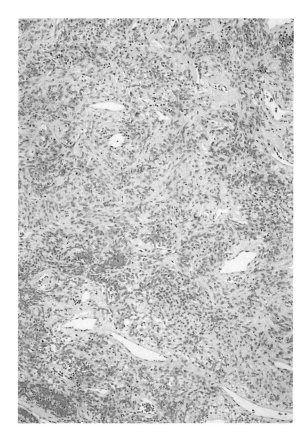

Figure 6-4
LOCALIZED FIBROUS TUMOR OF THE PLEURA
This pattern of growth is characteristic.

features of these areas are similar to those seen in parts of some desmoplastic DMMs. A stori-form pattern of distribution may also be seen and can cause confusion with sarcomatous mesothelioma (fig. 6-5).

Cellular areas composed of closely packed spindled or oval cells of varying size and scant intervening stroma may be found in more than half of the tumors (fig. 6-6). In these cellular areas, interdigitating fascicles may be formed. A small number of tumors are uniformly cellular. Mitoses (2 to 15 per 10 high-power fields) and nuclear pleomorphism may be present in these cellular areas, and in less cellular areas as well (fig. 6-7). Some mimic hemangiopericytoma, particularly in cellular regions (fig. 6-8) (6).

Foci of degeneration or cystic change occasionally occur in benign tumors. Areas of recent necrosis may be found in cellular neoplasms.

The pleura overlying the tumors generally shows fibrous thickening, but the adjacent meso-thelium is inconspicuous. Usually the surface appears denuded of its mesothelial layer, although focally a single layer of plump mesothelial cells may be seen in well-preserved specimens (fig. 6-9). In tumors attached to visceral pleura, epithelial structures of papillary or tubular form have been observed frequently. Foster and Ackerman (11), who believed these elements were of mesothelial origin, found them in 8 of 18 cases and noted that they lay near the periphery of the tumors (11). We have observed that in tumors that project deep into the lung substance, the tumor boundary often contains spaces lined by a single layer of cuboidal or low columnar epithelium of respiratory type. Cleft-like spaces lined by this epithelium sometimes dip into the tumor substance (fig. 6-10). These findings, along with the absence of

103

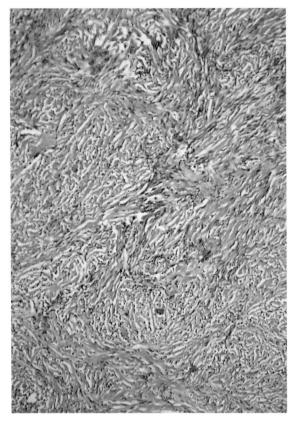

Figure 6-5
LOCALIZED FIBROUS TUMOR OF THE PLEURA
A storiform pattern is seen.

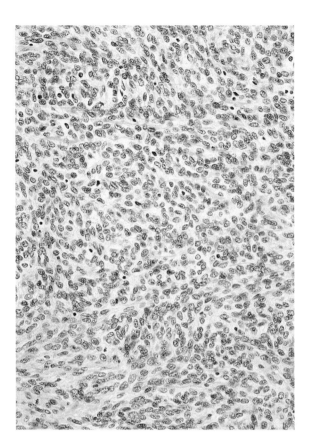

Figure 6-6
LOCALIZED FIBROUS TUMOR OF THE PLEURA
This cellular area has a predominance of oval cells.

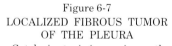

Figure 6-7
LOCALIZED FIBROUS TUMOR
OF THE PLEURA
Cytologic atypia is seen in an other-
wise benign localized fibrous tumor.

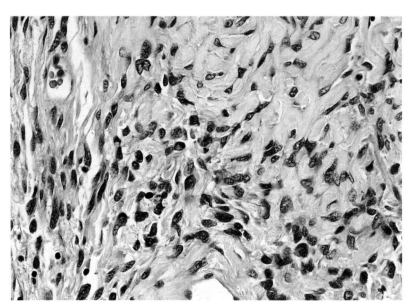

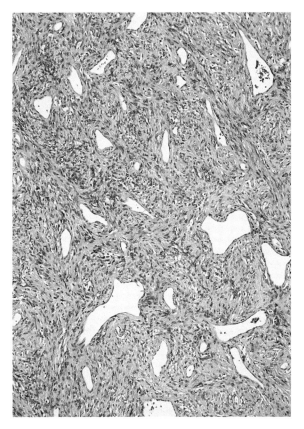

Figure 6-8
LOCALIZED FIBROUS TUMOR OF THE PLEURA
An area mimicking hemangiopericytoma.

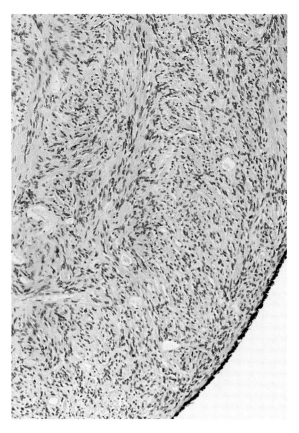

Figure 6-9
LOCALIZED FIBROUS TUMOR OF THE PLEURA
The tumor cells do not immunoreact when immunostained with antibodies to low molecular weight cytokeratins. However, the surface layer of mesothelial cells is intensely stained.

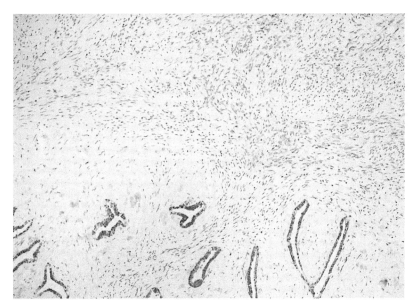

Figure 6-10
LOCALIZED FIBROUS TUMOR OF THE PLEURA
Deeper portion of the same tumor shown in the previous figure. The tumor cells do not immunoreact when immunostained with antibodies to low molecular weight cytokeratins. However, many cleft-like spaces lined by metaplastic epithelium express cytokeratin.

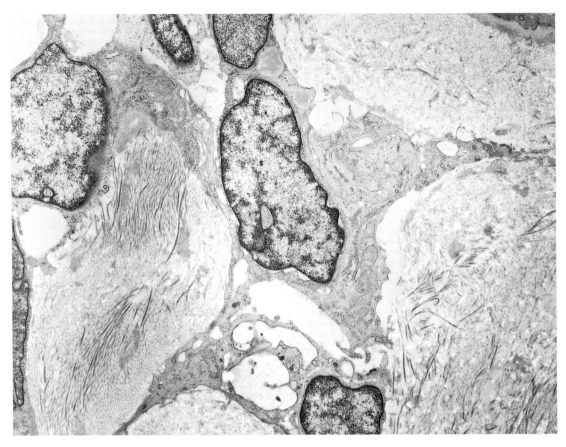

Figure 6-11
LOCALIZED FIBROUS TUMOR OF THE PLEURA
Electron micrograph of a typical example of localized fibrous mesothelioma. The tumor cells lack distinctive ultrastructural features.

epithelial components in the deeper portions of the tumor, or in the proximity of the pleura, indicate that the epithelial component of localized fibrous tumor of the pleura usually represents inclusions of non-neoplastic bronchiolar or alveolar epithelium.

Electron Microscopy. Ultrastructural studies are few and have sometimes been applied to tumors in unusual anatomic locations or that are malignant. Most observers have found that cells of either fibroblastic or undifferentiated type predominate (fig. 6-11) (3,13,27), but others have seen cells with the characteristics of fibroblasts and mesothelial cells (8,16).

Immunohistochemical Findings. Most authors report absence of expression of cytokeratins or other epithelial markers by the spindle cells of localized fibrous tumor of the pleura (figs. 6-9, 6-10) (4,5,7,10,23). These observations

support the nonmesothelial origin of the cells of this tumor. The absence of expression of cytokeratins may be useful in distinguishing it from sarcomatous mesothelioma (4,5,19). It was recently reported that a large proportion of localized fibrous tumors of the pleura express CD34, an antigen present in hematopoietic progenitor cells, normal endothelium, and a variety of vascular neoplasms (fig. 6-12). Sarcomatoid mesothelioma, on the other hand, lacks expression of this molecule. Using cytokeratin and CD34 antibodies in combination is highly effective for distinguishing these two entities (22).

Diagnosis and Clinicopathologic Correlation. In the classic situation of a tumor projecting from serous membrane into the pleural cavity as a polypoid mass of fibrous character, the diagnosis of localized fibrous tumor of the pleura is usually straightforward. More difficult

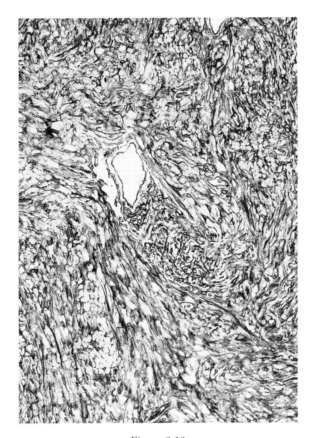

Figure 6-12
LOCALIZED FIBROUS TUMOR OF THE PLEURA

All the tumor cells, as well as the endothelial cells, are strongly reactive when immunostained with a monoclonal antibody to CD34 antigen.

to classify is the tumor that lies mainly in the lung substance or chest wall, especially when it is cellular or vascular. The histologic appearance of such tumors often overlaps that of various soft tissue tumors. It has been noted that intrapulmonary tumors of pleural origin are of anaplastic spindle cell type (25) and that intrapulmonary spindle cell tumors with visceral pleural involvement have a relatively high grade of malignancy, as compared with localized tumors found only in the pleural space (12). However, others have found that malignant characteristics are not more prominent in deeply situated growths (11). Local recurrence or metastasis following resection has been reported in a small number of more superficially located localized fibrous tumors of the pleura. We found that 6 of 37 tumors (16.2 percent) that were not entirely

intrapulmonary recurred and that 5 (13.5 percent) metastasized (6). Similar experience has been reported by others (20). England et al. (10) recently reviewed 223 cases of localized fibrous tumors of the pleura clinicopathologically. In this large series, 82 (37 percent) were classified as histologically malignant based on the presence of high cellularity, more than 4 mitoses per 10 high-power fields, pleomorphism, hemorrhage, and necrosis. Nonetheless, 45 percent of the tumors deemed to be malignant were cured by simple excision. Indeed, in this series, resectability was the most important indicator of clinical outcome. Other factors that correlated with malignant behavior were: tumors arising from parietal, mediastinal, or interlobar fissures and tumors arising in the visceral pleura that had an "inverted" growth pattern into peripheral lung rather than a pedicle.

In some series, malignant-behaving tumors expressed cytokeratins, raising the possibility that they were histogenetically different neoplasms (22). Evidence of malignancy usually appears within 1 or 2 years, but, rarely, may be delayed for many years (6,20). Metastases may sometimes be widespread and involve tissues and organs such as liver, bone, skin, adrenal, and the opposite lung and pleura (6). Local recurrences, however, often have a benign histologic appearance (20,26).

The presence of a supporting pedicle and resectability in general are considered to be the best indicators of good prognosis (3,10). Malignant tumors are generally larger than 10 cm in diameter at the time of surgical resection and are cellular in most areas (6,10). Mitotic activity is usually present and sometimes 10 or more mitoses per high-power field are seen. Cytologic atypia, although infrequent, may be considerable in malignant examples (fig. 6-13), and foci of necrosis are frequently seen (fig. 6-14).

Treatment. Many polypoid pleural tumors have been treated by simple resection, without taking significant amounts of lung tissue. However, the frequency of local recurrence with this tumor should encourage a more extensive resection (20). Wider resection of lung tissue is clearly desirable when the tumor is partly or mainly intraparenchymal. There is no evidence that radiation is effective in tumor control.

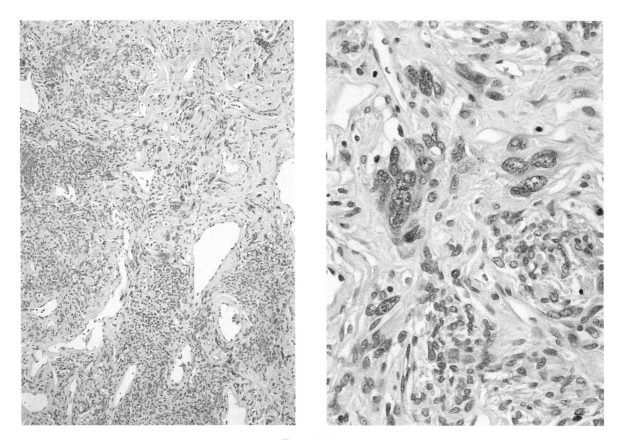

Figure 6-13
LOCALIZED FIBROUS TUMOR OF THE PLEURA
Otherwise typical, this example had several foci of highly atypical, cytologically malignant cells.
Left: An area of transition from typical fibrous tumor to an atypical component.
Right: Larger magnification of highly atypical, malignant-appearing cells.

Figure 6-14
LOCALIZED FIBROUS TUMOR
OF THE PLEURA

A large area of ischemic necrosis is
seen in this typical case of fibrous
mesothelioma.

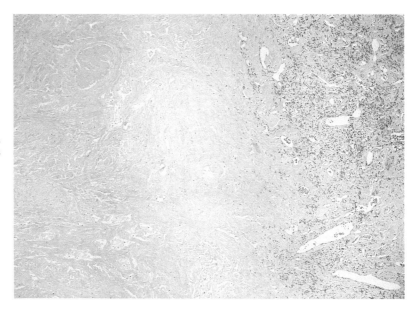

REFERENCES

1. Al–Izzi M, Thurlow NP, Corrin B. Pleural mesothelioma of connective tissue type, localized fibrous tumour of the pleura, and reactive submesothelial hyperplasia. An immunohistochemical comparison. J Pathol 1989;158:41–4.

2. Andrion A, Mazzucco G, Bernardi P, Mollo F. Sarcomatous tumor of the chest wall with osteochondroid differentiation. Evidence of mesothelial origin. Am J Surg Pathol 1989;13:707–12.

3. Briselli M, Mark EJ, Dickersin GR. Solitary fibrous tumors of the pleura: eight new cases and review of 360 cases in the literature. Cancer 1981;47:2678–89.

4. Cagle PT, Truong LD, Roggli VL, Greenberg SD. Immunohistochemical differentiation of sarcomatoid mesotheliomas from other spindle cell neoplasms. Am J Clin Pathol 1989;92:566–71.

5. Carter D, Otis CN. Three types of spindle cell tumors of the pleura. Fibroma, sarcoma and sarcomatoid mesothelioma. Am J Surg Pathol 1988;12:747–53.

6. Dalton WT, Zolliker AS, McCaughey WT, Jacques J, Kannerstein M. Localized primary tumors of the pleura: an analysis of 40 cases. Cancer 1979;44:1465–75.

7. Dervan PA, Tobin B, O'Connor M. Solitary (localized) fibrous mesothelioma: evidence against mesothelial cell origin. Histopathology 1986;10:867–75.

8. Doucet J, Dardick I, Srigley JR, van Nostrand AW, Bell MA, Kahn HJ. Localized fibrous tumour of serosal surfaces. Immunohistochemical and ultrastructural evidence for a type of mesothelioma. Virchows Arch [A] 1986;409:349–63.

9. El–Naggar AK, Ro JY, Ayala AG, Ward R, Ordóñez NG. Localized fibrsous tumor of the serosal cavities. Immunohistochemical, electron-microscopic, and flow-cytometric DNA study. Am J Clin Pathol 1989;92:561–5.

10. England DM, Hochholzer L, McCarthy MJ. Localized benign and malignant fibrous tumors of the pleura. A clinicopathologic review of 223 cases. Am J Surg Pathol 1989;13:640–58.

11. Foster EA, Ackerman LV. Localized mesotheliomas of the pleura. The pathologic evaluation of 18 cases. Am J Clin Pathol 1960;34:349–64.

12. Guccion JG, Rosen SH. Bronchopulmonary leiomyosarcoma and fibrosarcoma. A study of 32 cases and review of the literature. Cancer 1972;34:836–47.

13. Hernandez FJ, Fernandez B. Localized fibrous tumors of the pleura: a light and electron microscopic study. Cancer 1974;34:1667–74.

14. Ibrahim NB, Briggs JC, Corrin B. Double primary localized fibrous tumours of the pleura and retroperitoneum. Histopathology 1993;22:282–4.

15. Kauffman SL, Stout AP. Mesothelioma in children. Cancer 1964;17:539–44.

16. Kay S, Silverberg SG. Ultrastructural studies of a malignant fibrous mesothelioma of the pleura. Arch Pathol 1971;92:449–55.

17. McCaughey WT. Primary tumours of the pleura. J Pathol Bacteriol 1958;76:517–29.

18. _____, Dardick I, Barr JR. Angiosarcoma of serous membrane. Arch Pathol Lab Med 1983;107:304–7.

19. Montag AG, Pinkus GS, Corson JM. Keratin protein immunoreactivity of sarcomatoid and mixed types of diffuse malignant mesothelioma: an immunoperoxidase study of 30 cases. Hum Pathol 1988;19:336–42.

20. Okike N, Bernatz PE, Woolner LB. Localized mesothelioma of the pleura: benign and malignant variants. J Thorac Cardiovasc Surg 1978;75:363–72.

21. Ratzer ER, Pool JL, Melamed MR. Pleural mesotheliomas. Clinical experiences with thirty-seven patients. Cancer 1967;99:863–80.

22. Renshaw AA, Pinkus GS, Corson MC. CD34 and AE1/AE3. Diagnostic discriminants in the distinction of solitary fibrous tumor of the pleura from sarcomatoid mesothelioma. App Immunohistochem 1994;2:94–102.

23. Said JW, Nash G, Banks-Schlegel SP, Sassoon AF, Shintaku PI. Localized fibrous mesothelioma: an immunohistochemical and electron microscopic study. Hum Pathol 1984;15:440–3.

24. Stout AP. Tumors of the pleura. Harlem Hosp Bull 1952;5:54–57.

25. _____, Himadi GM. Solitary (localized) mesothelioma of the pleura. Ann Surg 1951;133:50–64.

26. Utley JR, Parker JC Jr, Hahn RS, Bryant LR, Mobin-Uddin K. Recurrent benign fibrous mesothelioma of the pleura. J Thorac Cardiovasc Surg 1973;65:830–4.

27. Wang N. Electron microscopy in the diagnosis of pleural mesothelioma. Cancer 1973;31:1046–54.

28. Witkin GB, Rosai J. Solitary fibrous tumor of the mediastinum. A report of 14 cases. Am J Surg Pathol 1989;13:547–57.

29. Young RH, Clement PB, McCaughey WT. Solitary fibrous tumors ("fibrous mesotheliomas") of the peritoneum. A report of three cases and a review of the literature. Arch Pathol Lab Med 1990;114:493–5.

30. Yousem SA, Flynn SD. Intrapulmonary localized fibrous tumor. Intraparenchymal so-called localized fibrous mesothelioma. Am J Clin Pathol 1988;89:365–9.

31. Zukerberg LR, Rosenberg AE, Randolph G, Pilch BZ, Goodman ML. Solitary fibrous tumor of the nasal cavity and paranasal sinuses. Am J Surg Pathol 1991;15:126–30.

7
SECONDARY TUMORS OF SEROSAL MEMBRANES

A wide range of tumors, especially carcinomas, may spread to serous membranes. Serosal metastases follow direct extension from adjacent viscera, transcoelomic dissemination, or permeation of underlying lymphatics. Often it is obvious from the clinical and pathologic evidence that the serosal deposits are metastatic. Sometimes, however, the clinical features and histologic appearance makes distinction from mesothelioma difficult.

PLEURA

Carcinoma of the lung is the most common cause of malignant pleural effusion (17). Peripheral carcinomas often extend to the visceral pleura. Usually, involvement is localized to the area immediately overlying the tumor, but, occasionally, neoplastic seeding of the pleural surfaces and confluent sheets or masses of tumor are seen. Any histologic type of lung cancer may involve the pleura, but adenocarcinoma is the most common because of its frequent peripheral location. The primary tumor may be overshadowed by the pleural-based growth in some cases (fig. 7-1), and the term *pseudomesotheliomatous adenocarcinoma* has been proposed for such cases (6,10,16). Peripheral lung cancers resembling bronchiolar carcinoma have a particular propensity to imitate mesothelioma (10), but oat cell carcinoma and other histologic types may do so as well, albeit rarely. Adhesion to the parietal pleura and involvement of the chest wall or vertebral column may follow. The so-called Pancoast's tumor (superior pulmonary sulcus tumor), in which a carcinoma at the lung apex involves nerves in the root of the neck, is an example of this extension.

Carcinoma of the breast is the most common tumor to involve the pleura in women. Epithelial carcinomas arising in ovary, pancreas, thyroid, gastrointestinal tract, and kidney often seed the pleural surfaces as well. This seeding is frequently coupled with, and probably often secondary to, tumor permeation of subpleural lymphatics. The surface tumor deposits are usually in the form of multiple granulations or nodules on the visceral pleura, but, occasionally, areas of diffuse pleural thickening result. Metastatic renal cell carcinoma occasionally presents with a clinical picture mimicking pleural diffuse malignant mesothelioma (DMM) (29). We have seen two cases of sarcomatoid renal cell carcinoma involving the pleura that clinically and radiologically mimicked mesothelioma; distinguishing them from sarcomatous mesothelioma was not possible either histologically or immunohistochemically.

Malignant lymphomas and leukemias are the third most common category of tumor causing pleural effusion (17). Chylous effusions are especially likely to be associated with lymphoma (23).

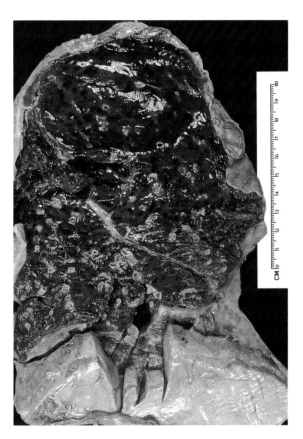

Figure 7-1
PSEUDOMESOTHELIOMATOUS
ADENOCARCINOMA
Extensive involvement of the pleura by an adenocarcinoma arising at the lung periphery. The gross and radiologic picture is indistinguishable from that of diffuse pleural mesothelioma. (Courtesy of Dr. Hidejiro Yokoo, Chicago, IL.)

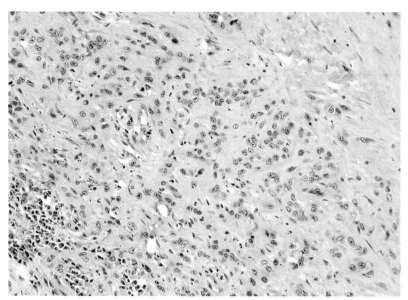

Figure 7-2
EPITHELIOID
HEMANGIOENDOTHELIOMA
This tumor presented with extensive pleural involvement causing it to be initially misdiagnosed as diffuse malignant mesothelioma. (Figures 7-2 and 7-3 are from the same case.)

The relative frequency of the histologic types of malignant lymphoma associated with effusions are about the same as those not associated with effusions (31). However, pleural effusion, and possibly pleural infiltration, appear to occur with increased frequency with lymphoblastic types (20) and with malignant lymphoma of peripheral T-lymphocyte origin (30). Pleural effusion may also occur in multiple myeloma and in some cases it is associated with myeloma infiltration of the pleura (12,15). Effusions due to metastatic cancer are caused by direct involvement of the pleura by tumor or by lymphatic obstruction leading to poor reabsorption of fluid. The latter mechanism is particularly common in lymphoma (31). Effusions caused by metastatic carcinoma and lymphoma are often bilateral. Bilateral effusions may also occur in bronchogenic carcinoma, especially when a mediastinal mass is present (22).

Sarcomas that metastasize to the lung or chest wall commonly involve the pleura and occasionally the pleural tumor predominates. The pleura may also be infiltrated directly by sarcomas arising in the subpleural tissues of the chest wall or lung and, rarely, such tumors progress to form a large mass in the pleural cavity. It may be difficult to determine the point of origin and histogenesis of these masses, especially when they are composed of undifferentiated spindle cells. Distinction from sarcomatoid mesothelioma may not be possible without immunohisto-

chemistry. Pulmonary epithelioid hemangioendothelioma arising near the serosal surface may extensively invade the pleura and mimic epithelial or biphasic mesothelioma clinically and histologically (fig. 7-2) (33). The use of appropriate immunohistochemical panels usually identifies these tumors (fig. 7-3) (2).

PERITONEUM

In western countries, the ovary is the most frequent source of metastatic carcinoma in the abdominal cavity, with the stomach, large intestine, pancreas, and breast being other common sources. The distribution of tumor deposits depends partly on the location of the primary, but the pelvic cavity is frequently involved. Commonly, the omentum is infiltrated at an early stage and later may be converted into a bulky and indurated mass. The mesentery and serosal surface of the intestine are other sites where tumor deposits are frequent. The nodular and confluent growth patterns that develop on the peritoneal surfaces are occasionally indistinguishable from those of DMM. The tunica vaginalis testis or the lining of a hernia sac may be involved by metastatic carcinoma, sometimes before the peritoneal tumor is clinically apparent.

The term *pseudomyxoma peritonei* (jelly belly) has been used clinically to describe the presence of masses of mucinous material in the peritoneal

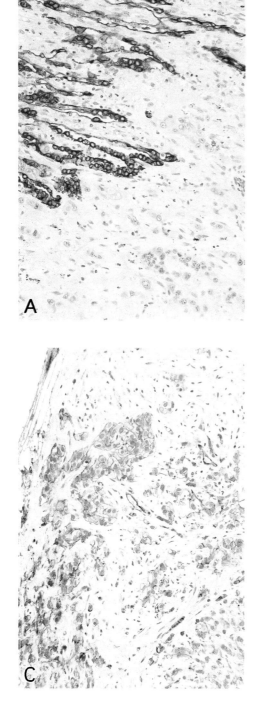

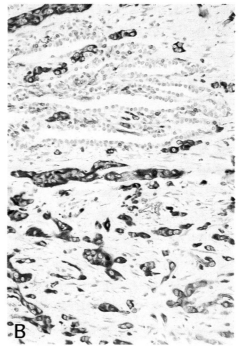

Figure 7-3
EPITHELIOID HEMANGIOENDOTHELIOMA

A: This section was stained with a cocktail of monoclonal antibodies to low molecular weight cytokeratins. There is strong immunoreactivity by the entrapped, irritated alveolar-lining cells but not by the tumor cells. This finding, in our experience, suffices to exclude the possibility of true mesothelioma.

B: This section was stained with a monoclonal antibody to vimentin. The alveolar cells (upper field) are minimally positive. The tumor cells are intensely reactive. This pattern (keratin negative, vimentin strongly positive) is common in hemangioendothelioma.

C: This section was stained with a monoclonal antibody to CD31. Strong, predominantly membrane-based staining of tumor and normal endothelial cells is present.

cavity, in association with a mucus-secreting tumor (mucinous cystadenoma or cystadenocarcinoma) in ovary, vermiform appendix, or as often observed, in both. The ovary has been considered to be the source of the peritoneal tumor, but often there is evidence supporting an appendiceal origin (32). Others hypothesize that the peritoneal tumor arises de novo as part of a multifocal neoplastic process (27). Tumor cells may be sparse or absent in biopsies of mucinous material and may sometimes appear benign or of low-grade malignancy. Patients in whom tumor cells are not found in peritoneal biopsies have a more favorable prognosis than those in whom tumor cells are present (32). It has been reported that intraoperative or spontaneous spillage of the contents of mucinous cystadenomas and borderline malignant mucinous tumors of the ovary does not lead to pseudomyxoma (9); others have noted widespread pseudomyxoma in association with benign and borderline mucinous tumors of the ovary (24,25). Recent additional evidence has supported the appendiceal origin of most cases of concurrent pseudomyxoma ovarii and appendiceal pseudomyxoma (21).

Patients with pseudomyxoma peritonei live from less than a year to a decade; most survive over 5 years (28). Repeated surgical intervention is the only therapy known to prolong survival (21).

Despite the absence of "destructive" stromal invasion in borderline malignant serous tumors of the ovary (ovarian serous tumors of low malignant potential), the peritoneal surfaces are involved by the tumor in 30 to 50 percent of cases (4). It is uncertain whether the peritoneal tumor represents seeding from the ovarian neoplasm or is autochthonous. The presence of an exophytic component in 70 percent of these ovarian neoplasms indicates a mechanism by which implantation might occur (19). The small size of the ovarian neoplasm in some instances, and the fact that serous cancers can develop in the peritoneum in the absence of ovarian involvement, makes a peritoneal origin plausible (5,8). In many cases the peritoneal tumor is superficial and noninvasive and is identical to the associated ovarian serous neoplasm in its striking papillary character, the presence of psammoma bodies, and the degree of epithelial hyperplasia (fig. 7-4). Superficial noninvasive tumor foci may also be associated with marked desmoplasia (3). When desmoplastic foci of tumor form between lobules of omentum they may simulate tumor invasion (see fig. 5-3). Invasive tumor is characterized by irregular infiltration of underlying tissue (fig. 7-5). Although borderline malignant ovarian neoplasms, by definition, are locally noninvasive, the accompanying peritoneal tumor frequently infiltrates. Infiltration and severe cytologic atypia correlate with an adverse prognosis (3,19). Rarely, the peritoneal tumor is composed of slender branching

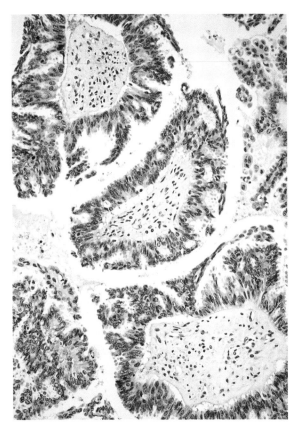

Figure 7-4
PAPILLARY SEROUS ADENOCARCINOMA
OF THE OVARY

This tumor diffusely involved the peritoneal surfaces and was associated with a primary ovarian tumor with a similar histologic appearance.

papillary fronds that are covered by a single layer of relatively uniform cells. Psammoma bodies usually occur with about the same frequency as in the associated ovarian tumor, although they may be much more conspicuous in the peritoneum because of associated fibrosis and lymphocytic infiltration (fig. 7-6). These bodies are also sometimes seen in the lumen and in the lamina propria of the fallopian tube. Benign-appearing epithelial lesions identical to those of endosalpingiosis sometimes accompany the peritoneal tumor (see fig. 5-4). In nearly 25 percent of cases of borderline malignant ovarian serous neoplasm with peritoneal lesions, endosalpingiosis is the only peritoneal abnormality (3). Endosalpingiosis may also occur in the absence of ovarian or other serous tumors and under these circumstances is frequently associated with chronic tubal inflammation (34).

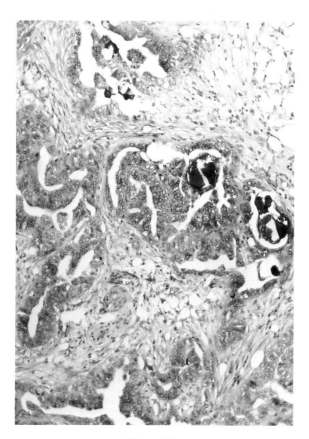

Figure 7-5
PAPILLARY SEROUS ADENOCARCINOMA
OF THE OVARY
Invasion of omentum.

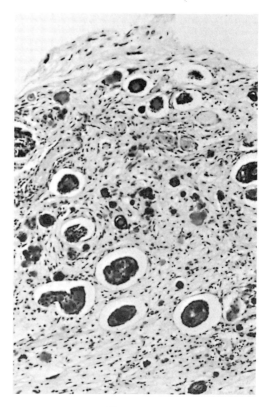

Figure 7-6
PERITONEAL PSAMMOMATOSIS
This peritoneal nodule shows numerous calcospherites dispersed through scar tissue. Shrunken epithelial cells surround most of the calcospherites. The patient had a borderline malignant ovarian serous papillary tumor and was found to have numerous peritoneal nodules of the type seen here (X120). (Fig. 119 from Fascicle 20, 2nd Series.)

Peritoneal involvement may adversely affect the clinical course of ovarian serous tumors of borderline malignancy, but are compatible with long survival. Over 50 percent of patients with stage IIb and III are well 5 years after diagnosis (13). Seven patients with peritoneal tumor who died had a mean survival of 8.9 years (14). There is evidence that the prognosis is closely linked to the character of the peritoneal tumor. The patients who die within a few years are generally those whose peritoneal tumor is histologically invasive at the time of initial surgery (5,19). We have not seen direct evidence of the progression of peritoneal endosalpingiosis to tumor, but the association of tumor with endosalpingiosis-like foci in some cases suggests that progression may occur. The development of tumor from endosalpingiosis in pelvic lymph nodes (Müllerian inclusions) has been described (7).

The most common source of metastatic serous papillary carcinoma involving peritoneum is the ovary but these carcinomas may also arise in the endometrium and share the tendency of their ovarian counterparts to spread over the peritoneal surfaces (11). Ovarian serous carcinomas present as disseminated intra-abdominal growths much more frequently than do their nonserous counterparts; this is probably because serous tumors tend to develop widespread focal carcinogenesis as opposed to a greater biologic aggressiveness (26).

Angiosarcoma and epithelioid hemangioendothelioma, as in the pleura, may diffusely involve the peritoneum. The gross and histologic features are similar to those of epithelial, papillary, or cystic mesothelioma (fig. 7-7).

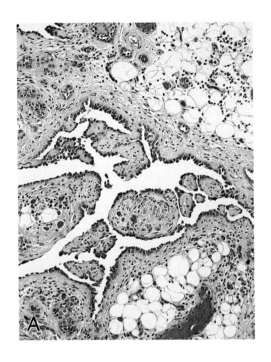

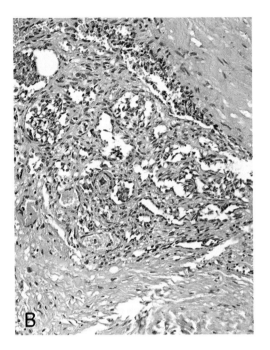

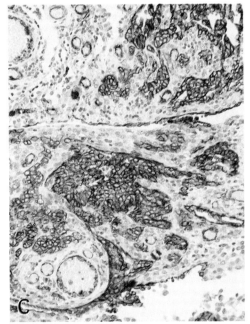

Figure 7-7
ANGIOSARCOMA OF PERITONEUM

Initially misdiagnosed as mesothelioma, this tumor features extensive superficial involvement of the peritoneal surface.

A: In many places the cells were columnar and formed papillary processes.

B: However, focal areas of typical angiosarcoma were found.

C: As in the case shown in figures 7-2 and 7-3, the tumor cells were strongly positive for vimentin and negative for cytokeratins. Additionally, they immunoreacted with several endothelial cell markers such as CD31, von Willebrand factor, and *Ulex europaeus.*

PERICARDIUM

Metastatic tumor to the heart frequently lodges in both myocardium and pericardium, but metastases from carcinomas of lung, breast, and thyroid, and sarcomas often involve the pericardium (18). Many tumors reach the heart by retrograde lymphatic spread, although the hematogenous route is also utilized, especially by sarcomas. Direct extension of tumor from adjacent viscera, such as lung, may also occur. Pleural mesothelioma often extends into the pericardium and when this occasionally occurs at an early stage, it is difficult to determine where the tumor originated. Malignant thymomas may also invade the pericardium by direct extension (1).

REFERENCES

1. Batata MA, Martini N, Huvos AG, Aguilar RI, Beattie E. Thymomas: clinicopathologic features, therapy, and prognosis. Cancer 1974;34:389–96.

2. Battifora H. Epithelioid hemangioendothelioma imitating mesothelioma. App Immunohistochem 1993;1:220–2.

3. Bell DA, Scully RE. Benign and borderline lesions of the peritoneum in women. Pathol Ann 1989;24:1–21.

4. _____, Scully RE. Serous borderline tumors of the peritoneum. Am J Surg Pathol 1990;14:230–9.

5. _____, Weinstock MA, Scully RE. Peritoneal implants of ovarian serous borderline tumors. Histological features and prognosis. Cancer 1988;62:2212–22.

6. Dessy E, Pietra GG. Pseudomesotheliomatous carcinoma of the lung. An immunohistochemical and ultrastructural study of three cases. Cancer 1991;68:1747–53.

7. Farhi DC, Silverberg SG. Pseudometastases in female genital cancer. Pathol Ann 1982;1:47–76.

8. Foyle A, Al-Jabi M, McCaughey WT. Papillary peritoneal tumors in women. Am J Surg Pathol 1981;5:241–9.

9. Hart WR, Norris HJ. Borderline and malignant mucinous tumors of the ovary. Histologic criteria and clinical behavior. Cancer 1973;31:1031–45.

10. Harwood TR, Gracey DR, Yokoo H. Pseudomesotheliomatous carcinoma of the lung. A variant of peripheral lung cancer. Am J Clin Pathol 1976;65:159–67.

11. Hendrickson M, Ross J, Eifel P, Martinez A, Kempson R. Uterine papillary serous carcinoma: a highly malignant form of endometrial adenocarcinoma. Am J Surg Pathol 1982;6:93–108.

12. Hughes JC, Votaw ML. Pleural effusion in multiple myeloma. Cancer 1979;44:1150–4.

13. Julian CG, Woodruff JD. The biological behavior of low-grade papillary serous carcinoma of the ovary. Obstet Gynecol 1972;6:860–7.

14. Katzenstein AL, Mazur MT, Morgan TE, Kao M. Proliferative serous tumors of the ovary. Histologic features and prognosis. Am J Surg Pathol 1978;2:339–55.

15. Kintzer JS, Rosenow EC, Kyle RA. Thoracic and pulmonary abnormalities in multiple myeloma. A review of 958 cases. Arch Intern Med 1978;138:727–30.

16. Koss M, Travis W, Moran C, Hochholzer L. Pseudomesotheliomatous adenocarcinoma: a reappraisal. Sem Diag Pathol 1992;9:117–23.

17. Leuallen EC, Carr DT. Pleural effusion. A statistical study of 436 patients. N Engl J Med 1955;252:79–83.

18. McAllister HA Jr., Fenoglio JJ Jr. Tumors of the cardiovascular system. 2nd Series, Fascicle 15. Washington DC: Armed Forces Institute of Pathology, 1978:52–8.

19. McCaughey WT, Kirk ME, Lester W, Dardick I. Peritoneal epithelial lesions associated with proliferative serous tumors of ovary. Histopathology 1984;8:195–208.

20. Nathwani BN, Kim H, Rappaport H. Malignant lymphoma, lymphoblastic. Cancer 1976;38:964–83.

21. Prayson RA, Hart WR, Petras RE. Pseudomyxoma peritonei. A clinicopathologic study of 19 cases with emphasis on site of origin and nature of associated ovarian tumors. Am J Surg Pathol 1994;18:591–603.

22. Rabin CB, Blackman NS. Bilateral pleural effusion. Its significance in association with a heart of normal size. J Mt Sinai Hosp 1957;24:45–53.

23. Roy PH, Carr DT, Payne WS. The problem of chylothorax. Mayo Clin Proc 1967;42:457–67.

24. Russell P. The pathological assessment of ovarian neoplasms. I. Introduction to the common "epithelial" tumours and analysis of benign "epithelial" tumours. Pathology 1979;11:5–26.

25. _____. The pathological assessment of ovarian neoplasms. II: The proliferating "epithelial" tumours. Pathology 1979;11:251–82.

26. _____, Bannatyne PM, Solomon HJ, Stoddard LD, Tattersall MH. Multifocal tumorigenesis in the upper female genital tract—implications for staging and management. Int J Gynecol Pathol 1985;4:192–210.

27. Sandenbergh HA, Woodruff JD. Histogenesis of pseudomyxoma peritonei. Review of 9 cases. Obstet Gynecol 1977;49:339–45.

28. Scully RE. Tumors of the ovary and maldeveloped gonads. Atlas of Tumor Pathology. 2nd Series, Fascicle 16. Washington, D.C.: Armed Forces Institute of Pathology, 1979:75–91.

29. Taylor DR, Page W, Hughes D, Varghese G. Metastatic renal cell carcinoma mimicking pleural mesothelioma. Thorax 1987;42:901–2.

30. Waldron JA, Leech JH, Glick AD, Flexner JM, Collins RD. Malignant lymphoma of peripheral T-lymphocyte origin: immunologic, pathologic, and clinical features in six patients. Cancer 1977;40:1604–17.

31. Weick JK, Kiely JM, Harrison EG Jr, Carr DT, Scanlon PW. Pleural effusion in lymphoma. Cancer 1973;31:848–53.

32. Young RH, Silva EG, Scully RE. Ovarian and juxtaovarian adenomatoid tumors: a report of six cases. Int J Gynecol Pathol 1991;10:364–71.

34. Yousem SA, Hochholzer L. Unusual thoracic manifestations of epithelioid hemangioendothelioma. Arch Pathol Lab Med 1987;111:459–63.

34. Zinsser KR, Wheeler JE. Endosalpingiosis in the omentum. A study of autopsy and surgical material. Am J Surg Pathol 1982;6:109–17

✧ ✧ ✧

8
NON-NEOPLASTIC LESIONS OF THE SEROSAL MEMBRANES

A number of non-neoplastic lesions involve the serous membranes. Some of these may grossly or histologically resemble neoplastic processes, particularly when they lead to fibrosis and mimic desmoplastic mesothelioma.

PLEURAL PLAQUES

Pleural plaques consist of discrete, raised, gray-white lesions which occur in the parietal pleura overlying the rib cage and diaphragm (fig. 8-1). They have a firm rubbery or cartilaginous consistency, but may also be stony hard because of heavy calcification. The surface can be smooth or nodular (fig. 8-2) and the edges tend to overhang. They vary in size from tiny "specks" to wide lesions, 6 cm or more in diameter (18). They are largely confined to the lower half of the pleural cavity and never involve the pleural apex. The superior surface of the diaphragm is commonly involved, often in the area of the central tendon (fig. 8-2). Less frequently, plaques may involve the pleural surface of the pericardial sac. Plaques on the lateral wall of the chest are often elongated and follow the line of the ribs.

The plaques consist of coarse, oligocellular collagenous connective tissue, the undulating fibers of which give rise to a coarse basket-weave pattern; some degree of calcification is often present. Although granulation tissue is not seen, fibrinous deposits may occur on the surface. Mesothelial cells are usually inconspicuous or absent. However, mesothelioma may be intimately associated with or even invade pleural plaques (fig. 8-3). Some lymphocytic infiltration may be observed at the deep margin of pleural plaques. The elastic lamellae in adjacent pleura often continue unbroken beneath the plaques, thus showing that the fibrosis is generated close to or at the serosal surface.

The association between pleural plaques and asbestos exposure has been amply confirmed by population studies and appears to be dose related (2). Their occurrence in talc workers is probably caused by asbestos contamination of most types of talc (25). Asbestos bodies are not seen within the plaques, but uncoated fibers have been found in ashed plaque tissue (10) and by electron microscopy (15). Plaques are probably formed as a result of asbestos fibers penetrating visceral

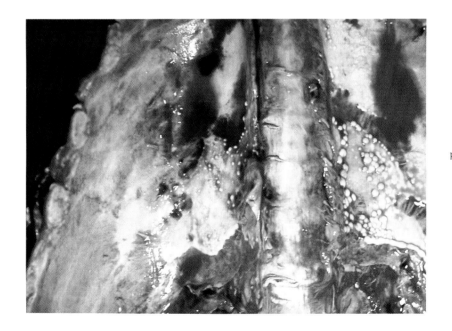

Figure 8-1
FIBROUS PLAQUE:
RIB CAGE
Typical aspect of fibrous plaque in an asbestos worker.

Figure 8-2
FIBROUS PLAQUE:
DIAPHRAGM
Dense, nodular, well-circum-
scribed plaque on the diaphragm
of an asbestos worker.

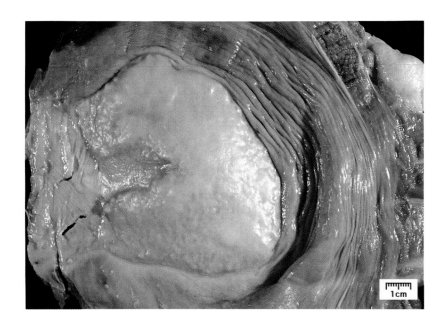

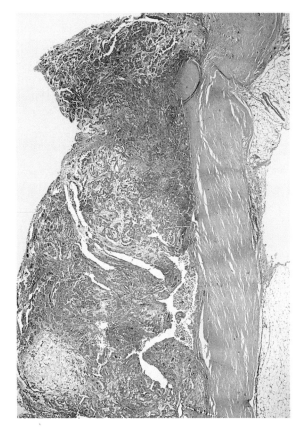

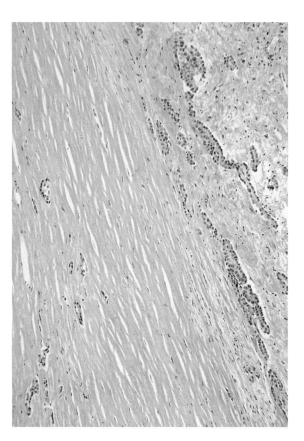

Figure 8-3
DIFFUSE MALIGNANT MESOTHELIOMA OVER FIBROUS PLAQUE
Left: The tumor is a typical epithelial type mesothelioma growing over the surface of the plaque.
Right: In some areas tumor invaded the plaque.

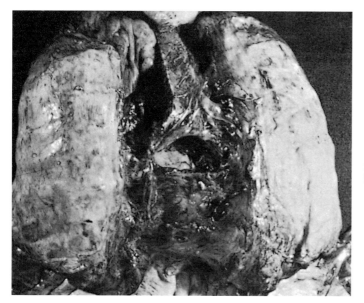

Figure 8-4
DIFFUSE PLEURAL FIBROSIS
IN ASBESTOSIS
The visceral and parietal layers of pleura were fused and thickened. (Fig. 124 from Fascicle 20, 2nd Series.)

pleura into the pleural cavity and being carried from there by the normal lymph flow to the parietal pleura. Once in the parietal pleura, the fibers are phagocytosed by macrophages which, in turn, release substances that stimulate submesothelial fibroblasts (9). There is no evidence of link between pleural plaques and the grossly similar lesion ("sugar icing") found on the surface of the spleen (24).

OTHER FORMS OF SEROUS MEMBRANE FIBROSIS

Diffuse thickening of the visceral pleura may occur in asbestosis (14) and the lungs may be encased, occasionally, by a thick layer of dense fibrous tissue (fig. 8-4). Extensive fibrosis may also occur in silicosis and, on occasion, in other forms of pneumoconiosis. Advanced hypersensitivity pneumonitis may be accompanied by prominent adhesive pleurisy, as may rheumatoid arthritis and, rarely, other connective tissue disorders. In the acute phase, rheumatoid pleuritis may be readily identifiable by its similarity to joint lesions and its characteristic cytology (7,20,31). Mostly, however, pleural fibrosis is a consequence of bacterial pneumonias, with the most marked examples occurring as a sequel of empyema.

Marked pleural fibrosis may sometimes be difficult to distinguish from tumor at the time of surgery or autopsy (11). Distinction from desmoplastic mesothelioma may be difficult even at the micro-

scopic level (see fig. 4-35) and may require immunohistochemical studies (see fig. 4-48).

The introduction of talc, starch, mineral oil, or other foreign substances into serous cavities may lead to the formation of nodules and adhesions. In the peritoneal cavity, such reactions have often been mistaken for metastatic carcinoma during surgery. Dense intestinal adhesions may follow any type of peritonitis and in patients with recurrent or chronic peritonitis, such as may occur with long-term peritoneal dialysis, widespread serosal fibrosis is particularly likely to develop. Peritoneal fibrosis may also occur in association with decompensated hepatic cirrhosis (4) and in patients treated with beta-adrenergic blocking agents (8,19).

Sclerosing (retractile) mesenteritis is a rare tumor-like lesion of the mesentery which is composed of chronically inflamed adipose and fibrous tissues in various proportions. There may be concomitant involvement of mesocolon, omentum, and retroperitoneal tissue, and intestinal adhesions. It is probably a nonspecific reaction to a variety of injuries (22).

CYSTS

The main type of cystic lesion that projects into the pleural cavity is an emphysematous bulla; occasionally, other types of peripherally located congenital and acquired cysts may abut the pleura. Mesothelium-lined cysts, including loose

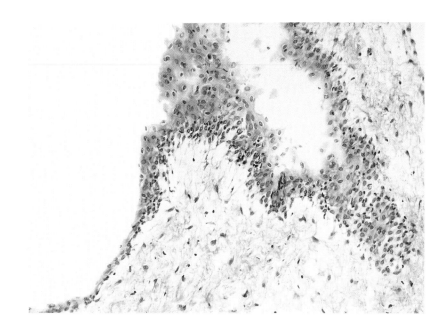

Figure 8-5
LOOSE PERITONEAL CYST
Cyst lining, showing a stratified, squamoid appearance.

cysts of the peritoneal cavity, have been described and occur mainly in women. These loose abdominal cysts may be single or multiple and range in size from 1.5 to 6.0 cm (14). Microscopically, they have a thin wall of connective tissue and are lined by cuboidal or columnar cells which may be stratified and squamoid (fig. 8-5). The so-called pericardial cyst is the most common cystic lesion associated with the pericardium and it is lined by mesothelial cells (16). These cysts are often attached to parietal pericardium and range between 1 and 15 cm or more in size.

ENDOMETRIOSIS

Endometriotic deposits are common in the peritoneum, particularly in the pelvic region. They are readily recognized by their red or bluish color. They may be difficult to diagnose in their later stages when fibrosis occurs or when present at unusual sites such as the pleura (23).

ENDOSALPINGIOSIS

This term refers to the presence of benign glandular inclusions of tubal epithelium outside the fallopian tube proper (28). Endosalpingiosis is widely believed to result from metaplasia of mesothelium, but the reported association with tubal damage has raised the possibility that it may be the result of implantation of tubal epithe-

lium detached by an inflammatory process (32). Though often not apparent grossly, it may occasionally be appreciated in the form of fine granularity or tiny cysts on the peritoneal surface (3).

The most common location is over the ovarian surface, close to the fimbria, suggesting that the condition may be secondary to inflammatory adhesions and overgrowth of tubal epithelium. However, endosalpingiosis may also occur with some frequency elsewhere in the abdomen, as is indicated by its presence in 16 of 128 surgical specimens of omentum from females (32). All of these patients had inflammatory tubal disease. The peritoneal lesions associated with papillary serous tumors of the ovary of borderline malignancy sometimes show features of endosalpingiosis.

The epithelial elements in endosalpingiosis, whether associated with ovarian tumor or not, may have a tubular, tubulopapillary, or papillary configuration. They are also sometimes accompanied by psammoma bodies (6,17,32). In some instances the degree of epithelial hyperplasia and atypia associated with a papillary or tubular formation is between that associated with endosalpingiosis and that found in borderline serous tumors. Such cases justify the designation *atypical endosalpingiosis*. Because psammoma bodies may be associated with endosalpingiosis it is important to remember that their presence in pelvic washings does not necessarily indicate cancer (5).

Endosalpingiosis may involve pelvic and para-aortic lymph nodes (Müllerian inclusions); the reported incidence in general autopsy and surgical material from females ranges from 5 to 14 percent (6).

LEIOMYOMATOSIS PERITONEALIS DISSEMINATA

Leiomyomatosis peritonealis disseminata (LPD) is a rare non-neoplastic multifocal proliferation of smooth muscle–like cells in the submesothelial peritoneal connective tissue. LPD is found mainly in women of reproductive age and is often associated with pregnancy or the use of contraceptive steroids (21,27,29,30). At laparotomy it presents as widely scattered multiple peritoneal nodules whose appearance often suggests metastatic tumor. Decidual tissue is sometimes noted in relation to the nodules and it seems that the condition is a result of fibrous replacement of decidua (21). However, the lesions of LPD have the characteristics of smooth muscle (30). Very

rarely, glandular tissue resembling endometrium occurs within the substance of the smooth muscle proliferations (13); also rare is adipocyte differentiation (12). It has been suggested that the LPD represents a hormone-induced metaplasia in submesothelial connective tissue (1,30), perhaps similar to that producing the decidual reaction that commonly involves this tissue in pregnancy. As the condition is benign and tends to spontaneously regress, a conservative approach to treatment is indicated (30). However, a case of LPD with malignant change has been reported (26).

Conditions that should be differentiated from LPD include leiomyosarcoma and benign metastasizing leiomyoma. The small size of the nodules of LPD and their immense numbers are unlike the findings in the latter conditions. Microscopically, LPD may be difficult to distinguish from benign metastasizing leiomyoma and differentiation is based mainly on the gross characteristics and distribution of the lesions (27).

REFERENCES

1. Aterman K, Fraser GM, Lea RH. Disseminated peritoneal leiomyomatosis. Virchows Arch [A] 1977;374:13–26.
2. Becklake MR. Asbestos-related diseases of the lung and other organs: their epidemiology and implications for clinical practice. Am Rev Respir Dis 1976;114:187–227.
3. Bell DA, Scully RE. Benign and borderline lesions of the peritoneum in women. Pathol Ann 1989;24:1–21.
4. Buhac I, Jarmolych J. Histology of the intestinal peritoneum in patients with cirrhosis of the liver and ascites. Am J Dig Dis 1978;23:417–22.
5. Chen KT. Psammoma bodies in pelvic washings [Letter]. Acta Cytol 1983;27:377–9.
6. Farhi DC, Silverberg SG. Pseudometastases in female genital cancer. Pathol Ann 1982;17:47–76.
7. Graham WR. Rheumatoid pleuritis. South Med J 1990;83:973–5.
8. Harty R. Sclerosing peritonitis and propanolol. Arch Intern Med 1978;138:1424–6.
9. Hillerdal G. The pathogenesis of pleural plaques and pulmonary asbestosis: possibilities and impossibilities. Eur J Respir Dis 1980;61:129–38.
10. Hourihane DO, Lessof L, Richardson PC. Hyaline and calcified pleural plaques as an index of exposure to asbestos. A study of radiological and pathological features of 100 cases with a consideration of epidemiology. Br Med J 1966;1:1069–74.
11. Kannerstein M, Churg J. Desmoplastic diffuse malignant mesothelioma. In: Fenoglio CM, Wolff M, eds. Progress in surgical pathology, Vol. II, New York: Mason Publishers, 1980:19–29.
12. Kitazawa S, Shiraishi N, Maeda S. Leiomyomatosis peritonealis disseminata with adipocytic differentiation. Acta Obstet Gynecol Scand 1992;71:482–4.
13. Kuo T, London SN, Dinh TV. Endometriosis occurring in leiomyomatosis peritonealis disseminata: ultrastructural study and histogenetic consideration. Am J Surg Pathol 1980;4:197–204.
14. Lascano EF, Villamayor RD, Llaur P. Loose cysts of peritoneal cavity. Ann Surg 1960;152:836–44.
15. LeBouffant L, Martin JC, Durif S, Daniel H. Structure and composition of pleural plaques. In: Bogovski P, Gilson JG, Timbrell V, Wagner JC, eds. Biological effects of asbestos. Lyon: IARC Sci Publ, 1973:249–57.
16. McAllister HA, Fenoglio JJ Jr. Malignant tumors of the heart and pericardium. In: Hartmann WH, ed. Tumors of the cardiovascular system. Atlas of Tumor Pathology, 2nd Series, Fascicle 15. Washington, D.C.: Armed Forces Institute of Pathology, 1978:77–8.
17. McCaughey WT, Kirk MR, Lester RW, Dardick I. Peritoneal epithelial lesions associated with proliferative serous tumors of ovary. Histopathology 1984;8:195–208.
18. Meurman L. Asbestos bodies and pleural plaques in a Finnish series of autopsy cases. Acta Path Microbiol Scand 1966;181(Suppl):1–107.

19. Morson BC. The peritoneum. In: Symmers WS, ed. Systemic pathology. 2nd ed. London: Churchill Livingston, 1978:1179–97.

20. Naylor B. The pathognomonic cytologic picture of rheumatoid pleuritis. The 1989 Maurice Goldblatt Cytology award lecture. Acta Cytol 1990;34:465–73.

21. Parmley TH, Woodruff JD, Winn K, Johnson JW, Douglas PH. Histogenesis of leiomyomatosis peritonealis disseminata (disseminated fibrosing deciduosis). Obstet Gynecol 1975;46:511–6.

22. Reske M, Namiki H. Sclerosing mesenteritis. Report of two cases. Am J Clin Pathol 1975;64:661–7.

23. Ripstein CB, Rohman M, Wallach JB. Endometriosis involving the pleura. J Thorac Surg 1959;37:464–71.

24. Robinson JJ. Pleural plaques and splenic capsular sclerosis in adult male autopsies. Arch Pathol 1972;93:118–22.

25. Rohl AN. Asbestos in talc. Environ Health Perspect 1974;9:129–32.

26. Rubin SC, Wheeler JE, Mikuta JJ. Malignant leiomyomatosis peritonealis disseminata. Obstet Gynecol 1986;68:126–30.

27. Tavassoli FA, Norris HJ. Peritoneal leiomyomatosis (leiomyomatosis peritonealis disseminata): a clinicopathologic study of 20 cases with ultrastructural observations. Int J Gynecol Pathol 1982;1:59–74.

28. Thor AD, Young RH, Clement PB. Pathology of the fallopian tube, broad ligament, peritoneum and pelvic soft tissues. Hum Pathol 1991;22:856–67.

29. Valente PT. Leiomyomatosis peritonealis disseminata. A report of two cases and review of the literature. Arch Pathol Lab Med 1984;108:669–72.

30. Williams LJ Jr, Pavlick FJ. Leiomyomatosis peritonealis disseminata: two case reports and a review of the medical literature. Cancer 1980;45:1726–33.

31. Yousem SA. Case for diagnosis. Multiple pulmonary rheumatoid nodules with an associated granulomatous pleuritis. Mil Med 1988;153:99,103–4.

32. Zinsser KR, Wheeler JE. Endosalpingiosis in the omentum: a study of autopsy and surgical material. Am J Surg Pathol 1982;6:109–17.

FUTURE DEVELOPMENTS

There is an average latent interval of about 35 years from the time of first exposure to asbestos to the development of mesothelioma, and most cases fit within the 20- to 50-year range. It is probable that the incidence of the tumor during the rest of this century has already been determined by industrial practices and environmental contamination that occurred 15 to 45 years ago. It also appears that there will be a continuing upward trend in the frequency of mesothelioma in some populations (3,4) although the magnitude of any overall increase remains speculative. Potentially adding to the long-term problem is commercial production in the past two decades of man-made fibers with nominal diameters of 1 μm or less (2). Outbreaks of malignant mesothelioma due to erionite fibers (1) and the experimental production of mesothelioma by glass and other nonasbestos fibers serves to warn of the carcinogenic potential of nonasbestos mineral fibers whose diameter and length are similar to asbestos fibers. In the future, diffuse mesothelioma may increasingly become a monitor of the carcinogenic effects of mineral fibers in general rather than just for asbestos. Through accurate diagnosis and classification, by stimulating inquiry into possible exposure to asbestos or mineral fibers in cases of diffuse mesothelioma, and by drawing attention to unusual frequencies and clusterings of the tumors, pathologists will have a continuing important role in the surveillance of this cancer. They have, and should continue to have, an expanding responsibility for investigation of the fiber burden of the lung and its composition.

Serosal neoplasms, including diffuse mesothelioma, can be accurately identified and classified in many cases using existing knowledge and routine staining techniques. However, the application of histochemical, and in particular, immunohistochemical techniques, will continue to permit more objective assessment in difficult cases and assist in earlier diagnosis. As evidence accumulates of significant differences in the biologic behavior of mesotheliomas of different histologic types, the importance of accurate histologic classification will increase. These developments should facilitate the application of promising forms of chemotherapy to the treatment of serosal neoplasms and more objective assessment of their results.

Increased recognition of precancerous atypical mesothelial hyperplasias and mesothelioma in situ presents interesting biologic and therapeutic challenges.

REFERENCES

1. Baris YI, Artvinli M, Sahin AA. Environmental mesothelioma in Turkey. Ann NY Acad Sci 1979;330:423–32.
2. Hill JW. Health aspects of man-made mineral fibres. A review. Ann Occup Hyg 1977;20:161–73.
3. McDonald AD, McDonald J. Malignant mesothelioma in North America. Cancer 1980;46:1650–6.
4. Newhouse ML, Berry G. Predictions of mortality from mesothelial tumours in asbestos factory workers. Brit J Industr Med 1976;33:147–51.

INDEX*

*Numbers in boldface indicate table and figure pages.

✧ ✧ ✧